# It's All in Your Head

## Everyone's Guide to Managing Concussions

Ann Engelland, MD

# Contents

# Foreword

The purpose of *It's All in Your Head* is to help anyone who has sustained a concussion, whether through playing sports, goofing around in a pillow fight, experiencing a motor vehicle accident, or tripping on the sidewalk. This book will help each of these victims and those around them to understand *right away* what their responsibilities and reactions need to be.

This book is intended to help injured people and those who care for them shortly after they get home following the injury. This may be within minutes to hours after the injury occurs or it may be after a trip to the ER or the hospital. It may also be many days after a concussion, or suspected concussion, has happened. Although head injuries evolve and the symptoms wax and wane and change, it is assumed that you are in a medically "stable" condition at the point of reading or listening to this book.

If you are unsure of whether your injury requires *immediate care right now*, turn to Chapter 5, Responding to What Just Happened for some guidelines and resources.

I chose to publish the book electronically because I want people to have immediate access to the information. It has become clear that the sooner the correct treatment is implemented, the faster and better the recovery from head injury and concussion will be. So with one, or maybe two, clicks, good, solid information and comforting stories and tips will be at hand.

## How this book was conceived

I am lucky enough to be a pediatrician and a school physician but also the mother of seven healthy and active teens and young adults. My interest in concussions began in the schools and through my patients, but my "research" began when I started talking to my children and their friends about the head injuries they have experienced but have never actually called a "concussion."

We sent out a Concussion Questionnaire to a circle of friends and from there this crowd-sourcing technique took on a life of its own. I have been astounded by the answers we received. I quickly realized that this book had to be written. Too many young men and women are continuing to play and are suffering without understanding what may have been wrong and how much risk they were bearing. The details they recounted about their concussions and the circumstances surrounding them are testimonies to our naïveté about the subject. The stories also reveal some aspects of our health care system and the role of sports in our culture and the impact of both of these on managing head injury.

*It's All in Your Head* is also meant to guide all of those surrounding the person who has had a head injury to better understand what the victim may be experiencing. Because it IS all in his or her head, nothing may be outwardly visible and he or she may be accused of faking or malingering and therefore be severely misjudged, misunderstood, or misdiagnosed. It is critical that everyone—parents, friends, teachers, work colleagues, coaches, bosses, therapists, tutors, and siblings—understand the ramifications of a concussion for the victim. If they do not, the treatment and rest required by the victim will be accelerated or skipped altogether and recovery could be prolonged, sometimes *indefinitely*!

That's right! It is possible to *not recover* from a concussion if the right steps are not taken. We think this way about heart attacks and strokes, don't we? It's time we started thinking this way about head injury as well. Concussions are very common and everyone in the community may experience a concussion some day, or be faced with someone who has suffered a concussion. Once you are enlightened, you will be able to help a victim recover successfully. Think of it as a new kind of CPR: Concussion Prevention and Response.

# Introduction:
## What Doctors Know Now

When I started out in pediatric practice I often took phone calls in the evening from parents with all sorts of questions about their children who were sick or had fallen or weren't sleeping. A typical call went something like this:

"Doctor, my son was jumping on the bed and fell off and hit his head. There's a big bump on his scalp. Could he have a concussion? What should I do?"

"How does he feel now?" I would ask.

"He seems fine. Maybe a little sleepy, but it's bed time."

"Did he pass out, even for a few seconds?"

"No, he cried right away and I put ice on the bump."

"OK," I would say, "he doesn't have a concussion then. I suggest you keep him awake for the next four to six hours and then wake him every two hours to check on him." Some doctors would even suggest shining a light in the child's eyes to check whether his pupils were "even" — as if parents really knew what that meant.

**We now know** that most of that advice was wrong.

Here's why:

- The *absence* of loss of consciousness does not rule out a concussion
- The *severity of a head injury* or concussion can not be judged at the time of the event
- If a person has a headache after a mild head injury the most important things to do are to *rest, be quiet, and sleep.*
- Allowing complete rest-both physical and cognitive (meaning *in the mind*)-is the right thing to do. Checking on a person is natural; *awakening* him or her is harmful.
- Shining a light in the eyes of a head-injured person is *not only annoying, but painful* and is likely to disrupt the healing process.

**So what is a concussion anyway?**

According to the Centers for Disease Control and Prevention, a concussion (officially called "minimal traumatic brain injury" or MTBI) is the occurrence of injury to the head arising from blunt trauma or acceleration/deceleration forces with one or more of the following:

**Any period of:**

- Transient confusion, disorientation, or impaired consciousness;
- Dysfunction of memory around the time of injury;
- Loss of consciousness

**Other observed signs following injury:**

- Seizures
- Irritability, lethargy, or vomiting, especially in young children
- Headache, dizziness, fatigue or difficulty concentrating, a befuddled look, unusual emotions, delayed reaction time.

❧

It's important to note what a concussion is NOT. It is NOT a bruise on the brain. It is does NOT show up on an X-ray the way a fracture or broken bone would. It does NOT have a blood test or other definitive examination to "rule it in or out," as doctors say. For the most part, it is defined by a constellation of these signs and symptoms many of which are subjective and depend on the patient's own story.

Medicine and first aid recommendations change all the time. How we respond to heart attacks and strokes has changed just as much in the past few decades as our response to head injury.

It's time that from children to the elderly, from students to superintendents, and from referees and first responders to doctors, we all get on board with how to Recognize, Respond, Rest, and Reassess possible concussions. Think of this as the Four Simple Rs.

Let's read on as we explore step by step how to do just that.

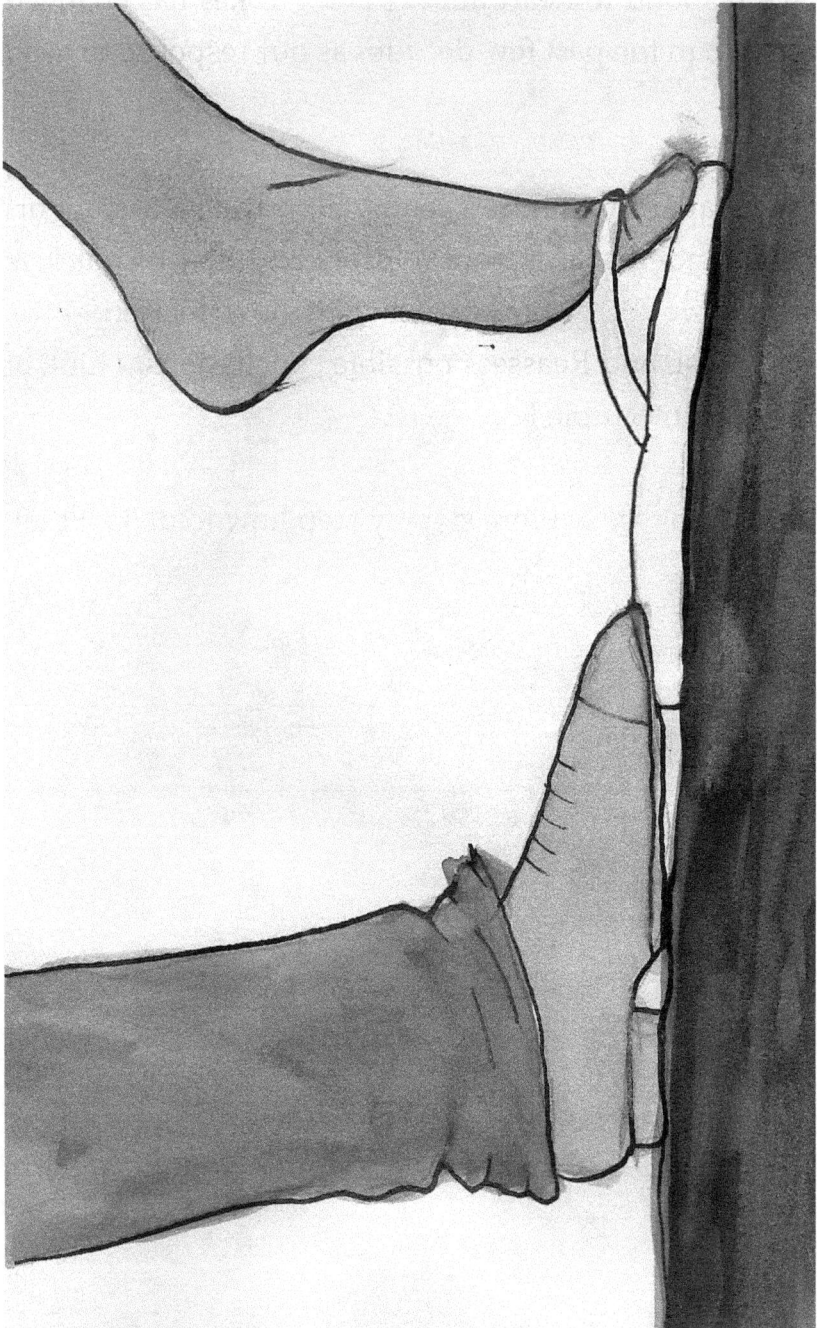

"I was walking down the street and I tripped and fell flat on my face."

# Chapter One:
## How It Can Happen

What follows are some vignettes from the questionnaires returned by athletes and friends who responded when asked if they had ever experienced a concussion. These snapshots illustrate the variety of ways that head injuries can happen. Sometimes people engage in activities in which head injury is part of the accepted risk. Other times, an injury occurs when least expected.

> *"When I was in my sophomore year of college, I had the unfortunate experience of being put through a ceiling. My friend was excited to see me and lifted me in the air and my head went through the ceiling, leaving a hole."*
> CS, age 19, female

> *"What I remember was riding the chairlift just before skiing and then waking up in the hospital. My father was with me and said it looked like I had simply taken a fall but when he came over to check on me there was a pool of blood and I was incoherent."*
> AJC, age 20, male

*"I was making a diving save while playing field hockey goalie and fell forward on my head. I got right back up and felt fine; just a bit dizzy for the rest of the game."*
KS, age 16, female

*"rugby game collision"*
NN, 31, with a history of at least ten "good ones", male

*"I injured myself in a horseback riding accident. While jumping, my horse's foot got stuck between two rails, and in a somewhat 'freak' accident, we both flipped over on the landing. I dove head first into the ground, and he rolled the other direction, luckily avoiding me."*
KAD, age 16, female, describing the first of two concussions

*"I was ice skating and my boyfriend lifted me up and then he put me down for a second so I would have a better grip, but when he lifted me up a second time, he lost balance on his skates while he was holding me. He dropped me and fell on top of me. I fell on my back and hit the back of my head against the ice."*
MN, age 17, female

*"I was playing football…My position was linebacker and I just led in with my head several times and got crushed."*
CS, age 15, male with a history of at least three concussions

*"…..running to a cab and tripped on my head fell head first on to the street in Manhattan. Had facial bruises and just a bit of pain in my head."*
OR, age 56, female

*"My last concussion was during a lacrosse game in 2001. It was my$2^{nd}$ concussion in as many months. I hit an offensive player at the same moment that he was following through with a shot…the momentum from my hit caused us both to hit the ground (him first on his back with my head whiplashing into his chest)."*
RNS, age 17, male

*"I was sitting in my airplane seat, without my seat belt on, and the plane (hit) some really rough, unexpected turbulence. I flew up out of my seat and hit my head pretty hard on the ceiling of the plane and came right back down into my seat."*
JF, age 17, male

*"I remember riding my bike slowly through an intersection. The next thing I remember was waking up lying on the street with someone gently shaking my shoulder. They told me they were putting me into an ambulance..."*
JH, age 31, male

*"Anna was shooting hoops with another girl (in gym class), practicing in advance of tryouts for the modified team. She decided to show off and throw up a shot and fade back... While most of the gym is padded, there are hoops on the sides and some of the walls behind them are not padded... Anna went back and hit the back of her head against the wall."*
AL, age 13, female (as recounted told by her mother)

ده

The Centers for Disease Control (CDC) in Atlanta, the U.S. government organization that tracks epidemiological data about all health-related matters in the United States, has compiled a great deal of data on concussions. Their statistics serve to illustrate the magnitude of the issue for our country. The CDC uses the term "Traumatic Brain Injury" or "TBI" in lieu of concussion. Among pediatricians and clinicians who manage sports-related head injuries, the term "concussion" still seems to be the most commonly used and the preferred word. TBI does, however, remind us that the issue at stake is the *brain!*

Figures from the CDC reveal that while the majority of TBI occur in the elderly, as many as a quarter of a million emergency room visits are made annually for sports and recreation-related concussions among children and adolescents. Experts believe that large numbers of head injuries never make it to an emergency room or into the data system. The answers to our questionnaire bear this out. Many of our respondents said that they had never seen a doctor or had a formal diagnosis for their injury.

As concussion awareness increases, the numbers of visits to doctors, outpatient clinics, and emergency rooms will undoubtedly go up.

Most of us who care about children, athletes, and patients with head injuries would interpret a temporary increase in the number of reported concussions as a good thing. That would mean that more people are becoming aware of the seriousness of their injury and getting the advice they need to recover quickly and completely. Eventually, we hope that we will *prevent* some concussions and the numbers will decline.

But in the meantime, let's talk about how we can prevent the *worst* consequences that can result from a concussion.

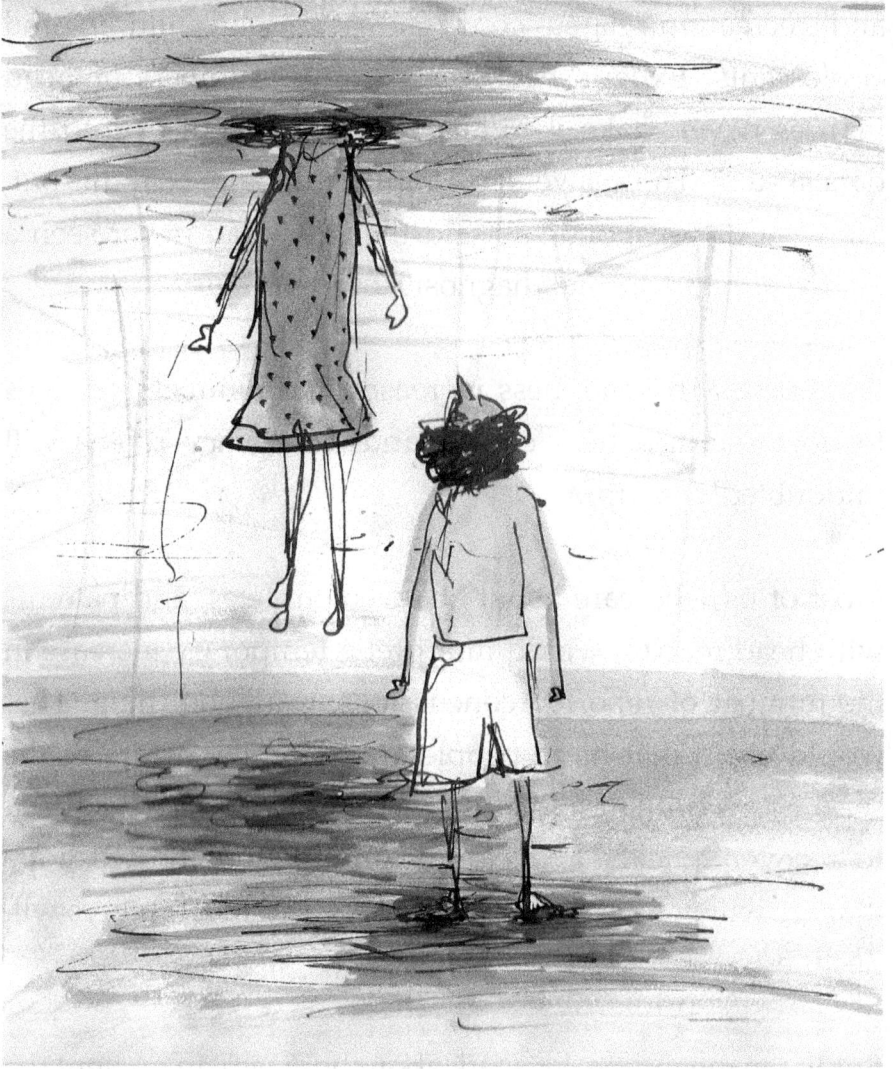

"My friend… lifted me in the air and my head went through the ceiling, leaving a hole."

# Chapter Two:
## The Four Rs and the Four Ds

The premise of this book is that if we educate about and practice the Four Rs, we will prevent the Four Ds.

**The Four Rs are:**
**Recognize, Respond, Rest, and Reassess**

**The Four Ds are:**
**Dropping out, Depression, Dementia, and Death**

**The four Rs** — simple steps that we can expect every man, woman, or child to understand as first aid for the person who appears to have sustained a head injury. Or for the person who *might* have a head injury. And certainly for the victim who *clearly* has a head injury. Sometimes a head injury is obvious: there may be a lump on the head or the person may be bleeding from somewhere above the neck. And sometimes a serious accident or episode has just occurred but there is no *obvious* head injury. In either situation, immediate action should be taken.

Many people know the Heimlich maneuver, as illustrated

by that poster near the restroom in most cafes, bars, and restaurants that demonstrates how to forcefully thrust on someone's abdomen to expel something that is causing him or her to choke.

And most people know to call 911 and suspect a heart attack when someone tells them an "elephant is sitting on their chest" and they can't breathe comfortably.

The hope is that eventually people will Recognize and Respond to head injuries in a similarly reflexive way.

# RECOGNIZE
**What do we mean by Recognize?**

Listen to the words of someone who had a concussion but didn't realize it:

> *"I got two concussions just from heading the ball. I tried to push through my initial symptoms thinking that I could do it...I was done."*
> SA, age 17, female, concussed playing soccer and had to quit all contact sports

*Choose life! Life is good! Go for it!*

We hear these expressions all the time, but in many situations we still choose to defy the odds. For example, we run a red light. We take risks. We think on the bright side of things. We ignore reality. We deny the facts. Often we get away with it. It's what makes some of us tick. It's what makes the world go round. And it's what has contributed to many of the world's greatest innovations.

In a 2012 NPR interview prior to the first Olympic women's boxing competitions, Vanessa Chakur, a former boxer, was asked about why women would choose to box and face the risks of head injury and chronic brain damage. "I loved exploring what was holding me back," she said. "I loved exploring my vulnerabilities, my weaknesses. I loved discovering strength I didn't even know I had." Shortly after this interview seventeen year old Claressa Shields went on to be the first ever American woman boxer to win gold at the Olympics.

But for most of us, on a daily basis, it's probably not a great idea to push the limits under all circumstances, and particularly when doing something that could result in a head injury.

First, it is critical to Recognize a head injury. Symptoms can vary, but here is a typical example:

*"It felt horrible...everything was a mirror image from earlier in the day; i.e., I felt like I was on the opposite side of the field and the mountains that were on the left were on the right, even though I was in the same place we started the day."*

CC, age 28, male

Immediate symptoms of a head injury may include:

- Confusion
- Dizziness
- Visual oddities
- Visual hallucinations
- Blackouts; loss of consciousness
- Headache
- Memory loss or amnesia

We will discuss these symptoms in more detail in Chapter Four: Recognize What Just Happened.

# RESPOND
**What do we mean by Respond?**

How we respond to a head injury depends on what the person was doing when the injury occurred.

For example, toward the end of the bicycling portion of a triathlon, two bikes collide and you go down. Your head is jarred as your body hits the pavement. You feel jangled. All shook up. You struggle to get back on the bike. You manage to shimmy through some narrow passages. You think you hear someone yell at you, unhappy that you have passed by too closely, but the sound is muffled. You manage to finish the race. You then stumble into your running shoes, feeling exhausted and sluggish. You begin running in the wrong direction. The course is not clear. You are escorted to the sidelines and you realize you have suffered a concussion. Now, you are forced to Respond.

Here's another example. Your daughter, Amanda, goes up for a header while playing soccer and collides with her opponent. You can almost hear their bodies crash. Amanda goes down and curls into a ball. Play is stopped and her teammates drop to a knee. Amanda, at first not moving, gradually pulls herself up to sit, holding her head. The coach pulls her out of the game and benches her. She sits still during half-time with her best friend's arm draped over her shoulder. To your surprise, coach sends her out to play in the second half. But she plays at half speed, misses a shot, and is subbed out after ten minutes of play. On the drive home all Amanda wants to do is sleep. You realize that she may have a significant head injury. You ask her if she thinks she had a concussion. Her answer surprises you: "Yes, probably."

"What is the right thing to do?" you ask her.

"Call the doctor?"

You are proud of her maturity but also feel nervous, knowing she must feel terrible.

After several questions from the doctor, the advice is to let her rest, check on her once or twice during the night but not wake her and not let her go to school the next day. So you put her to bed in a darkened room and let her sleep. She is grateful and sleeps most of the day. You give progress reports to her doctor and her coach.

The next day Amanda seems much better, but continues to sleep most of the day.

What about the Response in this situation? Frankly, it could have been better. *Amanda should not have played in the second half of the game.* She should have been benched for the rest of the game as soon as she was hit and showed symptoms of a headache, especially after a collision of such magnitude. Amanda recognized that her hit was significant and therefore her own response could have been more forceful and clear. As difficult as this can be for an athlete, Amanda should have let her coach know that she was not OK to return to play.

Recognizing and Responding to a head injury as quickly as possible is the best strategy to achieve the quickest recovery.

# REST
## What do we mean by Rest?

"Bed rest" is easier to imagine than to do. In the old days, doctors prescribed bed rest for all sorts of maladies, including rheumatic fever, tuberculosis, and pregnancy. Thankfully, for most people the days of bed pans and forced breakfasts in bed are over.

However, I have recently seen some pediatricians prescribe "bed rest" for patients with concussions in the hopes of forcing them to stay quiet. Listen to KAD, who was thrown from her horse and suffered a concussion at age 16:

> "The best advice I was given after my concussion was... to spend an entire week mostly in bed without looking at a single screen (phone, computer, television) and without reading. Essentially, I was told to make my mind do as little as possible. Though I was slightly bored, it was actually easy in my condition to spend all day sleeping or just lying in bed in a dark room with relatively little other activity."

"Rest" means absolutely no activity. This means no soccer, biking, hiking, or sports of any kind. It also means no working out, no walking, at first, and nothing else that might raise the heart rate. No sex. No yoga. No dancing.

Got that? It's really pretty easy. Vegging out on the couch. Couch potato. Easy.

But what are you supposed to do while you "veg" out on the couch?

There's the problem.

Rest after head injury and concussion must include not only physical Rest but also cognitive Rest, or Rest for the mind.

This is one of the major differences between the management of concussion now and even in the recent past. We now recognize that the work of the brain includes all of the functions of the brain and that all of the intellectual activities (thinking, remembering, visual processing, organizing, analyzing, and learning) are affected by a concussion. All of these activities must slow down as much as possible in order for the brain to heal.

Boredom is the answer. That's right. **Boredom.**

For a short period of time you will be asked to be bored. Like you may never have been bored before. Like back in the days before phones, texting, Internet, TV, radio; even before pencil and paper. Hard to imagine, I know. But as you saw above, you may actually welcome this time because as soon as you push yourself, if you are honest, your head will hurt. Or if it doesn't bother you right away, it will a few hours later and you will realize that you have skinned that knee (your ailing brain) once again.

This may be the hardest part of recovering from a mild concussion. But if you have a mild concussion and you rest quickly and completely, it is very likely that you will heal quickly and completely as well.

But if you defy this simple rule, you may face a much longer recovery period and an even more dangerous time ahead. Before we discuss these complications, a brief word about the fourth "R": Reassess.

# REASSESS
**What do we mean by Reassess?**

Reassessment is the process of taking stock, of making sure that you are ready to move on to the next step in recovery. For some people this process moves quickly. Every day will feel better. And there will be steady improvement and progress will feel certain. For others, it will feel slow and may even seem to go backwards on some days.

Recuperation can be a moving target. Concussion recovery is very individual and can be unpredictable. But one thing is certain: the cornerstone of recovery is Rest for the brain and all of its functions. In today's fast-paced world this can mean a very frustrating and trying time. Your friends will be passing you by for a short time. Do not worry. You will be back on track soon. Chapter 9 will be dedicated to the process of figuring out when and how to get back to activities, sports, and life as you knew it before injury.

**So what are the Four Ds?**

Having introduced the Four Rs for recovery, it is worth mentioning those dreaded Ds, if only briefly.

**Dropping out?** What about that?

> *"I wanted to play college soccer. That had been my dream since I was a little girl. I had to take a medical leave from my high school and repeat my junior year."*
> SA, age 17, female, after three concussions in one season

SA's story illustrates a lack of awareness on her part and on the part of those around her at the outset of her injury that led to a very prolonged recovery period affecting her physical and academic performance. Ultimate recovery for her (which she *has* achieved) depended on the support of a loving family and strong psychological support from her high school, family, and health care providers. Her own competitive personality and drive helped to get her through the highs and lows and achieve emotional and physical recovery.

## Depression?

In February 2011, Dave Duerson, a former NFL safety, aged 50, who had played with the New York Giants, Chicago Bears, and the Arizona Cardinals, shot himself in the chest after suffering depression and other serious issues. In a dramatic suicide text message he asked that his brain be sent to Boston University and studied for evidence of chronic neurodegenerative damage or chronic traumatic encephalopathy, thought to be caused by years of concussive impact to the brain. At autopsy it was indeed found that he did suffer from such neurodegenerative disease.

Unfortunately Duerson was not the first former professional football player to exhibit worrisome signs of brain damage. In November 2006, former NFL defensive back Andre Waters committed suicide after suffering from depression. Due in part to the persistence, intellectual curiosity, and a dedication to truth and justice for players by Alan Schwarz of the *New York Times* and others, the extent of the legacy of years of trauma-inducing play is beginning to come to light.

## Dementia?

Dementia is a frightening condition and unfortunately there is compelling evidence that recurrent brain injury and concussions can lead to brain damage that is similar to, but distinct from, Alzheimer's disease. The Sports Legacy Institute in Boston was founded in 2007 by Dr, Robert Cantu, a neurosurgeon, and Chris Nowinski, a Harvard graduate, football player, and world-class wrestler, to study the diagnosis, prognosis, and prevention of brain disease in athletes who have suffered damage from chronic or untreated injuries.

Although their work began with the study of depression and dementia in athletes exposed to recurrent concussions or sub-concussive impacts, it has expanded to study the damage to injured veterans returning from wars in Iraq and Afghanistan, where they are often exposed to blast injury. The near future is sure to bring a flood of public information about this vitally important issue.

## Death?

Did you say death? Yes. Any one of these conditions — dropping out, depression, or dementia — can lead to or directly cause death. It would be naïve to separate the deaths that have made headlines from the head injuries that preceded them. We honor these victims and their lives by learning from their sacrifices, their tragedies, and their experiences.

Death, you might argue, is a rare and terrible side effect of playing sports or of falling off the bed or tripping on the sidewalk. True. But when concussions go unrecognized, people expose themselves to further injury. Sometimes these injuries are accompanied by symptoms that eventually get them off the field while other times the symptoms are too subtle to recognize. Regardless, a great deal of damage still happens beneath the surface.

**So let's maintain perspective and remember the reason for this book in the first place. It IS all in your head! You are generally the best judge of any injury you have sustained and also the best judge of when your recovery is going well. You are in the driver's seat.**

**Therefore, keep the Four Rs in mind and Recovery is very likely.**

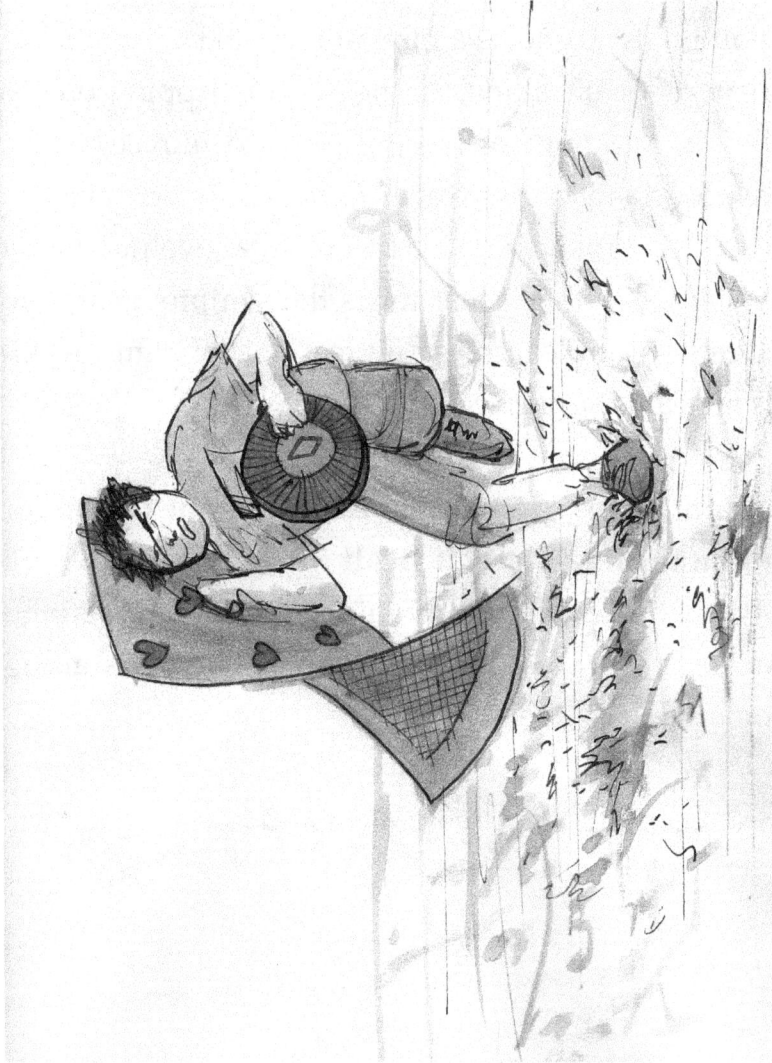

*"I remember telling (my rugby coach) that I was playing poker and what cards I was holding in my hand...."*

# Chapter Three:
## What We Want to Avoid

What we have learned over the past few decades is that there are essentially three important health conditions we hope to avoid by managing concussions carefully.

One of these is called *second impact syndrome*. It is rare but can be life-altering or lethal and has been the subject of numerous documentaries and videos that can be viewed by searching "Second Impact Syndrome" on the YouTube website, www.youtube.com.

The second condition, *post concussion syndrome*, is extremely common and has also been documented extensively. Indeed, millions of athletes play and millions of students study and learn with post concussion syndrome. Many of the respondents to our Questionnaire wrote about believing that they suffer from post concussion syndrome even months to years following their concussions. Many wonder if some of the problems they have are related to their prior concussions.

Most may never know the real answer to this because

so much of the damage to the brain can be quite subtle, muddled by other factors in life, and remains locked inside the cells and the architecture of the brain and unavailable to medical diagnosis at this time.

The third condition, **chronic traumatic encephalopathy**, and the one most recently recognized, is a form of cumulative and devastating neuropsychological impairment. For our growing understanding of this issue, we owe a debt of gratitude to the wives and families of many National Football League players for loving and caring for their ailing men who, it now turns out, were suffering from CTE.

Let's explore these three conditions in more detail:

**SECOND IMPACT SYNDROME: WHAT IS IT?**

*Second Impact Syndrome is a fatal or near-fatal swelling of the brain in a person who sustains a second concussion before a previous concussion has had a chance to fully heal.*

When this swelling occurs within a closed space (such as the skull) the inner structures are squeezed and irreversibly damaged, causing possible paralysis or even sudden death. Second Impact Syndrome is a rare event that is not well understood at a molecular or pathological level but when it happens on the field it can be devastating. No one knows how many cases of Second Impact Syndrome occur each year due to issues and controversies in reporting, but thankfully, the condition appears to be rare.

The devastating and dramatic nature of these Second Impact Syndrome events has caused schools to implement important changes in the way their communities handle concussions. In January 2012, CNN's Dr Sanjay Gupta interviewed a community where a Second Impact Syndrome death spurred change in North Carolina. This can be viewed through YouTube by searching for "Big Hits Broken Dreams."

While many of the changes and recommendations regarding Second Impact Syndrome have not yet withstood the rigors of scientific investigation, several committees of specialists have convened to create guidelines based on the group's best judgment and consensus.

Across the country, academic, hospital-based and community and state-level organizations and groups have begun to organize and create policies to direct and mandate schools, athletic programs and clinicians in the management of head injury. Almost all of these policies and recommendations are based on the simple principles of recognizing the subtle signs of concussion and teaching everyone to respond appropriately.

## POST CONCUSSION SYNDROME: WHAT IS IT?

Post concussion syndrome (PCS) is a constellation of symptoms that appear following a concussion or traumatic brain injury of any sort. According to UpToDate.com, a widely used and continuously peer-reviewed and updated website for physicians, symptoms of PCS include headache, dizziness, cognitive (or thinking) impairment, and psychological symptoms. The duration of the symptoms can be extremely variable. However, most patients recover within a few weeks. It is important to note that the duration and severity of PCS is not necessarily correlated with the *original and apparent* severity of the injury. An apparently mild hit or blow can require an unusually long recovery time. But another person, after the same "hit," might be symptom-free in only a few days.

Research has shown that early education and reassurance about what to expect right after the injury can make a big difference in the length of time that symptoms persist. As mentioned previously, recovery is a *process* that follows a forward moving, but often *unpredictable*, path, and each person is different. This "moving target" nature of recuperation challenges everyone, patients and clinicians alike.

We also know that Rest will shorten the time period until a person is symptom-free and also lessen the likelihood of symptoms lasting for weeks or maybe even years.

A key lesson here: If any activity causes symptoms—headache, dizziness, or unusual fatigue—the period of post concussion syndrome has not yet passed and Rest is still required. The brain is still healing.

The subject of post concussion syndrome has recently made national news. In May 2012, Kate Snow of NBC's *Rock Center* interviewed members of a girls' soccer team. Almost all of the girls had suffered multiple concussions and many were suffering from post concussion syndrome. The dramatic measures necessary (like living in darkened rooms) for their comfort begged the question of how and why these girls had been allowed by coaches, athletic trainers, and parents to play to the point of such severe brain injuries. The heartbreaking interviews during which they professed their love of the game, even at the expense of their academic and physical health, was almost too much to bear.

## CHRONIC TRAUMATIC ENCEPHALOPATHY: WHAT IS IT?

Chronic traumatic encephalopathy or CTE is a pathological condition—meaning it is described at autopsy. It was previously known as the clinical syndrome of *dementia pugilistica* because it was seen in fighters and boxers who showed signs of dementia, depression, and personality change late in life after a career in the ring. The association between fighters' brain disease and their head injuries is not new but it was only first described in the pathology lab and the term "chronic traumatic encephalopathy" or CTE, by which it is known today, was first coined in 1966.

It has become increasingly clear through the work of Cantu, McGee, and others at Boston University School of Medicine that there is a statistical and logical relationship between chronic head trauma and marked pathological changes in brain tissue. These researchers continue to pursue the study of the brains of football players and others with chronic head trauma.

How CTE actually develops is not yet fully understood but it is increasingly clear that there is a connection between persistent or unhealed brain injury and serious neurological and psychiatric symptoms such as *behavior and personality changes, depression, suicidal ideation, parkinsonism, speech abnormalities, and gait disturbances.* At autopsy, the brains of these athletes show atrophy, shrinkage, tangled brain matter, and a very particular type of protein deposit called "tau protein" in the superficial or outer layers of the brain.

Incontrovertible cause and effect proof of the link between repeated head injury and CTE may still be lacking and hard to get in a scientifically water-tight manner. However, public health and neuroscience experts are putting two and two together and making the *association* by listening to these stories. And unfortunately by seeing the end results in the injured brains of some who have died young or taken their own lives, they see that there are many ways the damage of concussion can manifest itself, sometimes many years after the initiating insults.

If you would like to listen to some poignant and striking stories from NFL wives who tell of the changes they noticed and lived with in their husbands you can hear them on YouTube. Search for NFL wives and concussions.

&

What we want to avoid following a head injury or concussion, then, is a range of problems from a headache that lingers for more than a few days and may be called *post concussion syndrome*, to the dramatic but rare complication of a *second impact syndrome* before the first concussion has fully healed, to the chronic and life altering brain changes of *CTE*.

All of these complications of concussion can result from hits that seem fairly insignificant at the time. Only by Recognizing a head injury for what it is and for its potential consequences can we avoid these problems.

# Chapter Four:
## Recognize What Just Happened

So you're all shook up.

Do you know what just happened? Could this be a concussion? Or is it just a "ding?" Did you get your "bell rung?" What does that mean, anyway?

Or is the most important thing the broken nose? Or getting back in the game? Or finishing the race? Or getting to the bottom of the slope? Or catching the bus?

No matter what else is going on, this short chapter will help you determine whether your injury may include a concussion.

Listen to the comments of these people who have had concussions and recall what it felt or looked like:

> "As I draw my stick back my peripheral vision fills up with white and it's not ice. There's no time to think. I send the puck sailing and brace myself. I close my eyes and BAMN (sic)! It's black. My eyes flutter open...but there's nothing

*routine about this one. I feel…off. I drag myself to the bench…I stumble in."*
Matt, age 14

*"My father said I thought I was ok and could ski down myself."*
AJC, age 20, rescued by ski patrol

*"I once got knocked out in a rugby game in Austin, Texas, didn't know the score, I was asking my teammate which direction we were headed on the field, my coach came out to talk to me, I remember telling him that I was playing poker and what cards I was holding in my hand. I ran around the field for another 5-10 minutes half dazed until they finally pulled me."*
NN, now age 31, never consulted a doctor about his concussions

*"I remember being in the ambulance and not being able to remember anything, including my name, which was the most frightening part."*
KAD, age 16

*"My head was throbbing uncontrollably and I lost color in my face and almost puked – granted, this was when I didn't know I had a concussion and worked out anyways…"*
EC, age 19

*"...seeing stars and overall confusion..."*
PS, age 17

*"For a full minute, I could only see the color yellow. I could hear, smell, touch normally – I was not unconscious – I actually stood up and tried to walk to the sideline; however, I could not see any images – just bright yellow. Once my vision returned, I became very nauseous."*
RNS, age 17

*"I took a kicked ball to the head. I lost memory for about two hours, went to the hospital and they did a CAT scan, not sure why, I don't recall anything for about 20minutes prior to the concussion to two hours after."*
XD, age 26

*"Right after the incident, I had a headache and experienced a little bit of dizziness. That was pretty much it. These symptoms subsided after about an hour or so."*
JF, age 17, hit head on airplane ceiling during turbulence

All of the above are possible **symptoms** of a concussion that a patient might report. A more complete list of symptoms includes:

Headache or pressure in the head
Nausea or vomiting

Balance problem

Dizziness

Double or blurry vision

Sensitivity to light or noise

Feeling sluggish, hazy, foggy, or groggy

Concentration or memory problems

Confusion

Just not feeling "right" or feeling "down"

(According to the CDC Heads Up program; June 2010)

In addition to **symptoms**, there are also **signs** of a concussion, meaning abnormal findings that a trained observer such as a trainer, EMT, coach, health care provider, or educated parent or bystander might observe in someone who has sustained a head injury. Signs of concussion include:

Appears dazed or stunned

Confused about assignment or position

Forgets an instruction

Unsure of game, score, or opponent

Moves clumsily

Answers questions slowly

Loses consciousness (even briefly)

Shows mood, behavior, or personality changes

Can't recall events prior to injury

Can't recall events after injury

## It's All In Your Head

(According to the CDC Heads UP program; June 2010)

If you are an athlete and are playing with a trained coach, trainer, or other professional on the sidelines, you may be evaluated using a tool called the SCAT 2, short for the Sport Concussion Assessment Tool 2.This tool is available as a free app as well. It does require some practice to administer it, score it, and interpret it efficiently. Although you may be tempted to try some parts of the test at home, do not do so if you have just suffered a head injury as your results may not be accurate and may cause your symptoms to worsen. Not what the doctor ordered!

Let's go back to dings and bell ringers. What are they, anyway?

According to the Urban Dictionary, when it comes to sports, having your bell rung "refers to when a player undergoes such a huge blow to his head that he can hear a ringing noise in his head." A "ding" is more or less the same thing.

Back in the days of macho play, when coaches would send their players right back in to play no matter what just happened as long as they were still standing, it didn't matter if the players were experiencing any signs or symptoms of concussion. But now that we can measure brain function through neurocognitive testing (more about that later), it has been shown very clearly that even when a player "just has his bell rung" or merely sees stars, it still may take up to a week for reaction times and short- term memory functions to return to baseline. So the important thing is to stop and Recognize that these mild injuries may really be more important than we used to think.

Since this chapter is about Recognizing what just happened there is a tool that you will find useful to help determine whether you have some of the symptoms and signs of concussion that we have just talked about. It is called the Symptom Checklist and it is in the Appendix of this book.

Here is what you can do within the first 24-72 hours following your injury to help decide if you may be dealing with a concussion whether in yourself or in someone you care about:

- Read the Symptom Checklist in the Appendix.
- If you are the injured person, HAVE SOMEONE READ THE LIST TO YOU.
- Determine your score.
- Don't be surprised if the score is very high.

After a head injury many people may experience symptoms on this checklist that they don't even attribute to a concussion. "Oh, I thought that was just sort of a hangover from the two beers I had last night. Even though two beers never gave me a hangover before." That kind of rationalization happens all the time because people are not aware of all the aspects of brain function, which we will discuss more in Chapter Six.

*It is important to determine your symptom score as soon as possible after an injury. That way you will be able to measure your own progress over the following days and weeks by using this simple tool. It is also very possible that your score will increase before it improves. Be patient and in the meantime, Rest.*

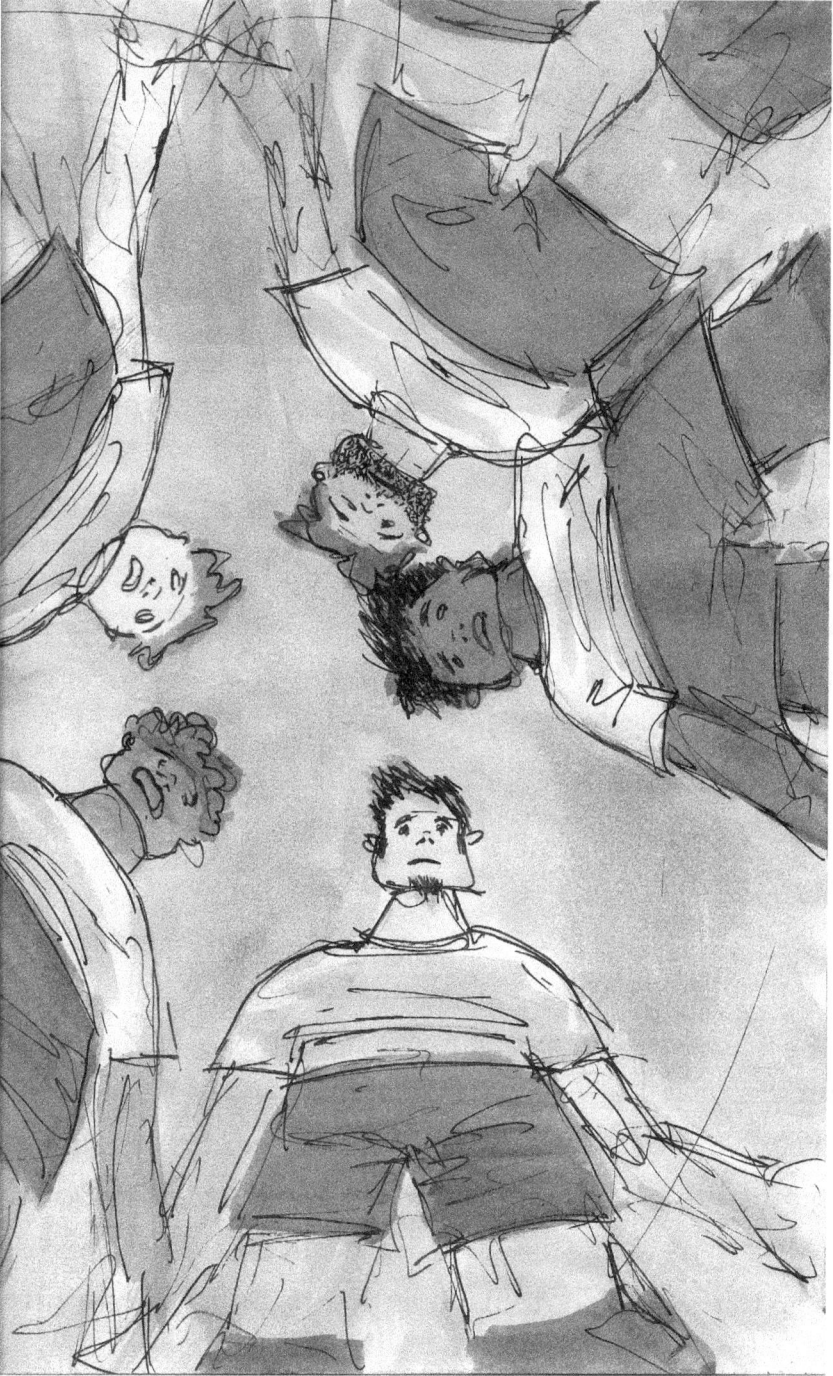

"First thing I remember was my team looking down at me"

# Chapter Five:
## Responding to What Just Happened

How do we know when the situation warrants high tech intervention, sirens, emergency response, ambulances, CT scans, neurologists and maybe even more?

Great question! Let's answer it right now because we need to get that one out of the way since this book is for the overwhelming majority of folks who do not have an *immediately* life-threatening emergency. The kind of threat to life we are talking about in *It's All in Your Head: Everyone's Guide to Managing Concussion* is a threat to quality of life, possibly a life-long one.

The first things to be concerned about in any injury are the ABC's. Airway, Breathing and Circulation. These decisions are made at the moment of injury by coaches, referees, certified athletic trainers, EMT's and other first responders. If you have come home from the game, even if you have made a trip to the ER, you have already passed Go and are extremely likely to have an injury in the "non-urgent" category.

If you did make a trip to the emergency room there is a strong possibility that you have had a CT scan or even an MRI. Experts argue about the appropriateness, necessity and cost effectiveness of these expensive studies. Expert guidelines exist to help health care providers make these decisions, but once a patient reaches an emergency room, the studies are often ordered "just to be sure."

Whether a CT or MRI has been done or not and regardless of the results, the key to all head injuries, as with many illnesses and injuries, is careful follow-up.

Many will remember the tragic 2009 death of the actress, Natasha Richardson who apparently died of an epidural hematoma after what seemed to be a minor skiing accident. An epidural hematoma is a collection of blood between the skull and the brain often resulting from a skull fracture. In this type of rare brain injury it is not uncommon to feel insignificant symptoms for a brief period following the impact. One of the issues in her case may have been the delay (due to geography and other unknown factors) in getting Ms Richardson to appropriate medical care once she began feeling worse.

In general, *a worsening situation,* even after an ER or doctor's visit or "clearance" warrants a repeat visit or at least a phone call.

A worsening situation that would mean you should go to the Emergency Room (or *return* to the ER) would be marked by any of these symptoms according to the CDC website:

- Headache that gets worse and does not go away.
- Weakness, numbness or decreased coordination.
- Repeated vomiting or nausea.
- Slurred speech.
- Looking very drowsy or unable to be awakened.
- Having one pupil (the black part in the middle of the eye) larger than the other.
- Having convulsions or seizures.
- Inability to recognize people or places.
- Getting more and more confused, restless, or agitated.
- Having unusual behavior.
- Losing consciousness (*a brief loss of consciousness should be taken seriously and the person should be carefully monitored*).

෴

For the majority of people with head injuries, these dire symptoms and consequences are unlikely. But what we now know is that even mild injury requires correct Responses from the outset.

Changing the way we, as a culture, respond to head injuries is both difficult and necessary. We are a culture of competitors, fighters, champions; people who pick themselves up and "get back in the ring" or "get back on the horse" and have "stiff upper lips" and "keep our chins up" while we play through the pain. And it isn't just athletes who behave this way. All of us are taught to power through our ailments, take some more ibuprofen, put in our hours, and carry on.

Chris Lowinski, a world-class wrestler and now a founder of the Sports Legacy Institute, finally told someone he had sustained a concussion (one of many) during a fight after he experienced a throbbing headache and memory problems for weeks afterwards. Back in 2003 he was unaware that each time he had "seen stars" and had "double vision" he was actually experiencing a brain injury or concussion. Now an advocate, public speaker, and supporter of research to prevent concussions and change the rules of the game—literally—Chris still feels the effects of his injuries, and all due to his lack of knowledge at the time. Chris can be heard giving compelling testimony about his personal experience on YouTube.

This is how one football player in our Questionnaire responded to his injury:

*"I was tackled helmet to helmet by the hardest hitting player on the team. I was knocked out for a few seconds. Woke up on my back. Sat out the rest of practice and saw the trainer…I figured hits like that were normal."*
EP, age 16, male

Taking yourself out of the game is hard to do. So maybe you need to have some lines ready to use, if needed, before you are in a high-intensity competitive situation.

Try these lines. Each of them contains a "red flag" word (in italics) that should be taken seriously by a competent coach, certified athletic trainer, referee, parent or bystander. These lines are examples and they should get you out of the game immediately without too much push-back. But, they might actually require practicing ahead of time. You don't need to memorize them, but merely saying them out loud a few times will show you that it's possible:

"I really *took a good one*. I need to sit out."

"My *head hurts*. I need to sit out."

"I *hit my head*. I need to rest."

"I might have a *concussion*. I need a break."

"I *don't feel right in the head*. I can't dance anymore. Let me rest."

"My *vision is blurred*. I need to sit down. I need to rest."

"Please get me off the field. *Something isn't right*."

"I know I cut my forehead, but my *head really hurts*. Let me rest."

"I feel *dizzy and nauseous*. Maybe I have a concussion."

"I *can't think straight*. Please call an ambulance. Let me rest."

"I *feel mixed up*. I can't play anymore."

The hope is that it won't be long before the word "concussion" will cause most bystanders and professionals to Respond correctly. And by correctly, we mean to stop the play, activities, or whatever else is going on and respect the need to treat the head injury as an *emergency* that demands immediate care.

Most of the time the Response will not include stitches, an ambulance ride, expensive scans, blood tests, or much technology. It certainly won't involve CPR in all but the rarest of cases. At least not traditional CPR as in mouth-to-mouth breathing or chest compressions or the Heimlich maneuver.

But we might think of the right Response as a different kind of CPR — Concussion Prevention and Response.

It bears repeating that *all injuries can evolve into something more although most do not.* The potential for this evolution is one more reason that the correct Response after a head injury or even a suspected head injury is to withdraw from play or activity.

Trust your instinct. And remember: It's all in your head.

# Chapter Six:
## The Human Brain

Since a concussion is also known by the scary term "Minimal Traumatic Brain Injury" or MTBI, maybe we should stop and consider all of the things or tasks the **brain** actually does, because each of these tasks that we might take for granted is affected by a concussion.

If we don't understand all the ways an injury can impact the brain, we might overlook symptoms that are actually indicators of an ongoing healing process. As we saw in Chapter Four on *Recognizing* a concussion, sometimes the symptoms and signs of a concussion can be quite subtle. And we have also seen that jumping back to activities before the brain is ready can delay healing or even lead to a second concussion.

I like to divide the tasks of the brain into five categories:

- **Motor (or physical)**
- **Cognitive (or intellectual)**
- **Emotional (or feeling)**

- **Psychological**
- **Social**

**What are motor tasks?** They include the following:

Walking
Balance
Gait (the style of your walk)
Coordination
Reaction time
The senses: Vision, Hearing, Taste, Smell, Touch

> *"Balance and the ability to sprint and run without a headache was tough."*
> RD, age 26, male

> *"...was quite sensitive to noise and loud sounds and fast images on TV..."*
> OR, age 56, female

**What are cognitive tasks?** They include the following:

- Reasoning
- Processing of new information (learning)
- Memory, both short- and long-term
- Organizational skills
- Ability to focus and concentrate

*"My memory is certainly not what it once was. Short term and long term."*
JH, age 31 at time of concussion

*"I had to work to remember short-term things for a few weeks but that all came back."*
RD, age 26

*"Later during that school year, AL started complaining of having trouble concentrating and kept insisting she had ADD."*
AL, age 13, as recounted by her mother

**What are emotional tasks?** They include the following:

- Moodiness
- Control of anxiety and worry
- Irritability
- Depression

*"Long term the biggest difference is that I started drinking again after being sober for a long time before my accident."*
JH, age 31

*"I was very emotional at the hospital and lost all my anger management control. I remember behaving erratically and was very upset and scared at the situation."*
KAD, age 16

*"I've battled depression in high school but I don't know if it was related to the concussions."*
EP, now age 29; sustained more than five concussions during high school

**What are psychological tasks?** They include the following:

- Regulation of drowsiness and alertness
- Sleep regulation

   *"Next day: stiff neck, felt tired, things were still cloudy."*
   EP, age 16

   *"The headaches in the following days, feeling confused — like cobwebs in my brain."*
   AJC, age 20

   *"The most important (symptom) to me was being in a fog for a week or two...Overall sluggish, but day-to-day tasks weren't overly effected (sic), just slower because of being tired and worn out."*
   PR, age 25

**What are "social" tasks?** They include the following:

- Judgment
- Following social cues

- Appropriate behavior in certain situations
- Manners (such as saying please, thank you, etc.)

*"...I've still got a headache creeping. I'm FINE! Screw this, I'm getting back out there. I'm patching up a boat with duct tape, spit and prayers, there's no way in hell I'm ditching my team because of a little pain. Maybe overconfidence, but it's killing me to sit on this bench..."*
ML, age 14, from a middle school essay describing his concussion during hockey

*"I was extremely emotional and depressed. Partly because the injury changed my brain functioning but also because the injury prevented me from doing the things I love: dancing and being social."*
LM, female, age 20; sustained two concussions within three weeks, first from a fall off the bed, then in dance class

One of the best and simplest explanations of what happens to the brain during a concussion is a six minute 2011 YouTube video by Dr. Mike Evans, a Canadian physician and "hockey Dad" who rapidly illustrates just how many of the brain's functions can run amok when a person has a concussion (key search words: Dr. Mike Evans, Concussion). I particularly agree with the premise of the brain as "mission control" and the image of the dumped-out file cabinets as a way of illustrating the disorganization often described as *fogginess.*

And Dr. Evans' lovely and unmistakable Canadian accent adds to the pleasure of this creative video.

# Chapter Seven:
## What Goes Wrong in the Concussed Brain

Most of our current understanding of what concussions are and the subsequent recommendations and clinical protocols on how to respond to them are based on experience and consensus among panels of experts. Not everyone will easily accept the changes that are being put forth for the rule books, on the fields, in clinics and in schools. As we have said before in this book, the culture of sports is a strong one.

But there continues to be fascinating work going on behind the scenes that is helping us gain a deeper and more objective understanding of what actually happens at a molecular and biological level to the injured brain. As a result there is increasing scientific data to back up these difficult recommendations.

This chapter is of a more technical nature and will briefly show that in laboratories, hospitals, clinics, and research facilities a great deal of work is going on in brain research at a molecular and anatomic level. If you are already convinced and/or not technically inclined, you can skip this chapter. But if you wish to learn a bit about the science behind the new understanding of concussion management, you may read on.

This chapter's brief lesson about the chemistry and biology of concussion is based on the work of scientists from many research institutions. Doctors Barkhoudarian, Hovda, and Giza at the Brain Injury Research Center at UCLA published a review article in *Clinics of Sports Medicine* in 2011 from which much of this information is paraphrased.

It is important to remember that a concussion is a *functional* disturbance and not a mechanical, anatomic, or otherwise visible abnormality. What this means, in practical terms, is that the *workings* or functioning of the brain are amiss. If the brain were your home, it might look fine, but when you flip the switch, the lights might not go on at all, or they might flicker or spark and then go out. In other words, the structure may appear fully intact, but the wiring is misfiring.

So what actually happens inside the concussed brain?

- A massive ionic imbalance takes place. Calcium, potassium, sodium and glutamate all shift in abnormal ways that contribute to inefficient neurons (these are the primary cells of the brain that conduct electricity and messages; i.e., are responsible for all functioning)

- There is a decrease in cerebral blood flow, meaning the delivery of blood and nutrients (primarily sugar or glucose, and oxygen)to the brain is diminished. It just sounds bad, and it is.

- The metabolism of glucose (or sugar, which is the brain's sole source of energy) is out of whack. Since glucose is the brain's only energy source, brain cells cannot use protein or fats from the diet. Therefore when the glucose machinery is malfunctioning, so is just about everything that the brain is responsible for.

- In a more severe head injury there can be swelling of the tissues in the brain and stretching of the axons (the long elegant tubules that conduct electrical signals between cells).

- Much work is being done now to study the effects of injury on what is called the "diffusion capacity" (essentially, the speed with which neurons can conduct messages). This appears to be affected in all injured brains, regardless of the patient's age. This is important information because until recently we have thought that young brains were more flexible and adaptable and could tolerate injury more readily. This may not actually be the case.

- Because of recent interest in and concern over the impact of chronic and recurrent injuries in certain sports, researchers are looking more closely at the protein deposits (tau proteins and others) that are being discovered in the brains of deceased professional athletes.

What researchers such as those at UCLA's Brain Injury Research Center and others have confirmed in the lab is that re-injury to an already damaged brain can have *a catastrophic metabolic effect*. This is the test tube or lab equivalent of second impact syndrome. As we discussed in Chapter Three, second impact syndrome on the field has been the impetus for so many of the revised policies now emerging around the country, and indeed the world, and changing the way we look at injury on and off the athletic field.

To summarize the relevant and important key points of the review article from UCLA's Brain Injury Research Center:

- Concussions can have both short and long term consequences
- After injury a sequence of events takes place that has immediate consequences on the functioning of the brain cells
- Injured brain cells have increased vulnerability to repeat injury for an ill-defined period of time
- Repeat injuries can be "seen" in behavior and

symptoms

- Repeat injuries can also be "seen" in brain tissue at autopsy
- Repeat injuries can be "seen" in living brains with some sophisticated kinds of scans that are not yet available to the general public
- Prevention of injury and particularly *prevention of repeat injuries* should be a major focus of public health efforts
- Adequate recovery time is critical for complete healing from any concussion injury in order to prevent repeat injuries that may have far more serious long term consequences than the initial one.

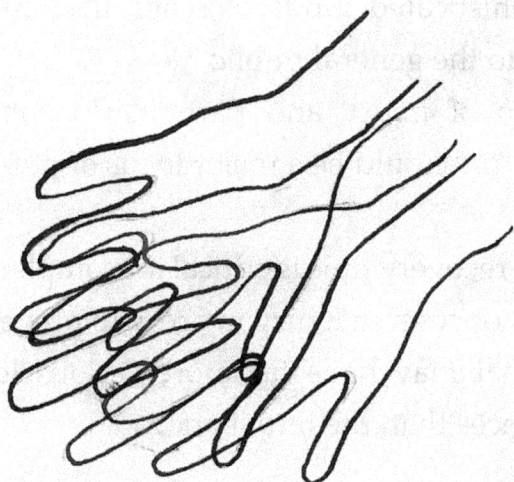

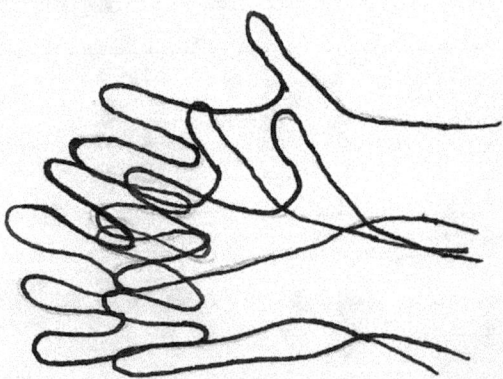

"I saw everything in double"

# Chapter Eight:
## What We Really Mean by Rest

As part of the Questionnaire (which you can read in its entirety in the Appendix of the book) we asked the question, "What kind of advice did you get about healing from your injury?" Questionnaire respondents reported receiving lots of advice to "take it easy" but very little specific advice beyond that. It is interesting to remember that most of these Questionnaire responses were sent to us at a time when the media was full of information about concussions and the importance of both rest and removal from play. Here were some of the responses we received:

> "I don't and didn't have health insurance. So they pretty much showed me the door and told me to rest up. I went back to have the stitches removed from my lips and tongue and really wasn't given any advice."
> JH, age 31, male, after being struck by a car

> "I was told not to fall asleep (my father actually stayed up with me and kept me from falling asleep). I was told to ice the back of my neck."
> EP, age 16, male, after football accident

*"Didn't get any advice."*
MB, age 29, male, injured in a rugby game

*"none"*
JD, age 16, male, soccer injury

*"...no alcohol, lots of water, no reliance on NSAIDS."*
DAR, age 25, male, rugby injury

*"...take pain killers; don't remember getting any others (advice)."*
KS, age 16, female, field hockey injury

*"The doctors told me I needed to wait at least a couple of weeks before returning to play. I had done research on the baseline testing and some of the other research around concussions at the time and decided to give myself plenty of time to heal. I hadn't had a baseline test done but wished I had."*
RD, age 26, male, rugby injury

The common thread among these stories is that only a few of the respondents were told to rest until they were symptom-free. Many were told to stay awake. The advice on "pain killers" varied widely. This is not meant to be an indictment of the doctors or other health care providers who offered this advice. It's possible that our respondents do not have complete recall of the advice given them. After all, memory is one of the casualties of concussion. Rather, these first-hand accounts serve to illustrate the need to establish simple and consistent advice for handling head injuries.

❧

As simple as it may seem, the cornerstone of treatment for most concussions is Rest. *A concussed brain cannot meet the energy demands of normal brain activities.* And as we have seen in the previous chapters, normal activities involve everything from sleeping, walking, talking, balance, and maintaining mood, to higher-order activities like thinking, organizing, solving math problems, and managing complex emotions. Taking a Rest from all of these activities will be necessary for a speedy and complete recovery.

For most people it will be important to enlist the help of friends, family, colleagues, school, and work to get through this phase of recovery.

**How long will this phase last?**

Recovery is extremely variable. Each person's injury is different and each person's recovery trajectory will be different. What seems to be true, however, is that the better the initial Rest period, the quicker the recovery. What does "better" rest mean? It means rest that is initiated as soon after the injury as possible and is as profound as necessary to prevent symptoms from flaring. Some people who suffer a concussion feel better within a week. Most will say they are back to normal within 2-3 weeks.

> *"Don't be tough, like you would with a bum ankle. Do not rush back until certain you are 100%."*
> PR, 25, male, assaulted; punched in head

How do I REST my brain?

When we talk about Resting the brain, we mean *physical and mental* rest. Post-concussion management used to just mean sitting on the sidelines and not playing. But even that is too much activity for many people. As one of our illustrations shows, it is possible to sustain injury just sitting innocently at a game. For many the noise and lights and fast action of a game can induce a post-concussion headache. In addition, we now know that the part we call **cognitive rest** is just as important as **physical rest**.

**Here is a list of things you should NOT DO in the days immediately following a concussion:**

- ✓ Drive
- ✓ Read
- ✓ Travel by airplane
- ✓ Play video games
- ✓ Watch TV (except *maybe* in short 10-15-minute

intervals)
- ✓ Use a mobile phone other than to listen
- ✓ Use a computer
- ✓ Text
- ✓ Have sex
- ✓ Do yoga (other than shavasana or the "corpse" pose)
- ✓ Exercise of any sort that raises your heart rate (this *may* include stairs and walking)
- ✓ Be around loud noises (this *may* include games and competitions with your team)
- ✓ Be around bright lights
- ✓ Be around physically jarring places (the subway, for example)
- ✓ Go on roller coasters

*"I had to turn the light on my phone and computer to a duller light b/c the light bothered my eyes and I stopped exercising for a month...I couldn't drive, go to school, and couldn't really leave my house."*
MN, age 17, female, dropped on head while ice skating recreationally

Many people who engage in the activities listed above following a concussion will develop a headache or feel unusually tired afterwards. *Pushing through that sort of discomfort is never a good idea.* The discomfort is a sign that the brain is not able to keep up and is not healed from its injury.

## So what CAN I do following a concussion?

For the first 24 hours, do as little as possible. Many people will want to sleep almost the entire time. It is part of the treatment to be BORED.

> *"That night I remember feeling an unusual urge to go to sleep and I had trouble focusing on my homework. However, at no point did my head hurt. Needless to say, the grade I received on my French test the next day was not great."*
> JD, age 26, male, recalling concussion sustained during soccer

> *"I was exhausted the entire week following the accident and spent most of the days sleeping. The week following my accident I stayed at home and slept. Within a week I was back on my feet and going about a relatively normal schedule, though I still had headaches and felt fatigued."*
> KAD, age 16, female thrown from horse

Once the need to sleep most of the day has passed, it is important not to push yourself back into regular activities too quickly. It becomes important at this point to actually **practice boredom!**

Things you CAN do (as long as they don't cause headaches):

- ✓ Rest, Rest, and Rest
- ✓ Listen to music
  - o One of my patients told me she found noise-reducing headphones particularly helpful
  - o Choose your genre of music carefully: some types may give you a headache
- ✓ Listen to books on tape
- ✓ Get a meditation tape from the library or off the Internet
- ✓ Daydream
- ✓ Have conversations
- ✓ Nap
- ✓ Invite friends over for short visits (one or two at a time to keep noise to a minimum)
- ✓ If you get a headache from visitors, let them know you have to cut it short
- ✓ Nap again

And of course you can EAT.

You must, in fact, eat. As with any healing process, your healing brain requires good nutrition. Even though you will not be exercising at all, your body requires healthy nutrients just to keep breathing and beating and sleeping and healing.

So some simple, common sense advice:

- ✓ Eat three good meals per day.
- ✓ Each meal should have some protein (meat, tofu, cheese, beans, or eggs).
- ✓ Do not overdo the sweet snacks. You will not feel like cooking so well-meaning friends may bring all kinds of junk. Limit your intake of junk.
- ✓ Drink plenty of water.
- ✓ Do **not** drink caffeine, alcohol, or other stimulant drinks (Red Bull, etc). These beverages will **not** help your headache.
- ✓ Eat five servings of fresh fruits and vegetables every day to keep your digestive tract healthy because you won't be moving around much. Constipation gives some people a headache; that's the last thing you want now.

**What about taking medication?**

You will undoubtedly have spoken to or seen your medical provider by this point. For the most part, if you are on regular medications you will continue to take those, but you should check with your doctor to be sure.

Following a concussion it is not advisable to take NSAIDs (non-steroidal anti-inflammatory drugs), more commonly known as the ibuprofen family of medications (brand names include Advil, Nuprin, Motrin, and many others) or drugs from the acetaminophen family, such as Tylenol.

Why?

Primarily because we do not want to mask the pain of a headache. *We want to know if the brain hurts* when doing certain activities. Pain is a major warning sign; a personal "wakeup" or, rather, "lights out" call that tells you that you need to REST! Go back to sleep. It's not time to be so active. Don't let yourself play through this pain. It will cost you in both the short and long run.

If you find that you cannot stand the headache or discomfort without taking medication, you should consult a health care provider. Sometimes prescription medications work better in a post-concussion situation. Rarely, a very bad headache is a sign of something more serious.

**How to help a friend with a concussion**

Your buddy or teammate or family member has sustained a concussion. Maybe you don't believe it. Maybe she doesn't believe it. Listen up: BELIEVE IT. There is no way to prove that someone has had a concussion. The only way for her to recover quickly and fully is to Rest. You can review Chapter

Two: The Four Rs and the Four Ds for a quick overview of the issues. But basically, here is what you need to do as a friend:

- ✓ Be quiet. Keep your voice down.
- ✓ Advocate for her: Let friends know that she cannot go to the game, the prom, the mall, the beach, the party, or work.
- ✓ Educate others about concussions. Concussions are common. One of their friends could be next. Everyone needs to learn and know the signs, symptoms, and treatment of concussions.
- ✓ Bring a playlist of quiet music. Suggest good genres to listen to.
- ✓ Read out loud (quietly) to her.
- ✓ Bring her a delicious salad to feed her brain.
- ✓ If she is ready to do homework, see how you can help.
- ✓ If she is a work colleague, let the boss and others know how she is doing. Advocate and educate at the workplace too. Have them download this book to learn more.
- ✓ If she is bored, figure out a way to encourage her to stay the course.
- ✓ When she returns to activities, have her back. If she doesn't look or act right, let her know. Everyone wants to deny symptoms. Staying home bored is not fun.
- ✓ Advocate for her even if she doesn't always do so for herself.

**When should I call the doctor?**

If a person has sustained a head injury and is clearly following the Rest protocol but is *getting worse in the first hours following the injury, he or she should be taken to the nearest emergency room as soon as possible.* This could be a life-threatening emergency requiring a CT scan or other evaluation and intervention. This was discussed in detail in Chapter 5: Responding.

Most school, college, and many athletic programs have developed protocols and programs to manage concussions which require the involvement of a physician or other health care provider to help manage the post-injury care of a concussed person. However, there are many people who experience "mild" concussions who never seek medical help or who do not return for evaluation because it is not required, not available, is unaffordable, or for other reasons.

Often a certified athletic trainer, school nurse, guidance counselor, or other professional who understands concussion can be a helpful partner and ally during the recuperation phase. I encourage any person with a concussion to seek help from a professional in his or her midst to be a sounding board and an advocate during the recuperation phase and to help reinforce the importance of true Rest.

If recovery is taking longer than a week and the patient does not seem to be on a *generally improving trajectory*, he or she may require a reassessment and should be seen by a health care provider. We will discuss this in the next chapter, Chapter Nine: Reassessing.

To summarize:

- Rest and boredom are the cornerstones of concussion treatment
- Too much activity will aggravate symptoms, primarily headache and fatigue
- It is difficult to predict how quickly an individual will recover fully
- Pushing the limits will delay recovery
- Stay in touch with your health care provider or other professional to create and stick with a game plan
- Enlist the help of friends and family to aid in your recovery.

# Chapter Nine:
## Reassessing

So at some point after your concussion, either the required waiting period will be up or you will just feel ready to try to advance beyond bed rest and get back in the ring. The key to progress is listening to *how you feel*.

As you recall, right after your injury YOU were the only one who really knew what was wrong inside. After all, it IS all in YOUR head.

For the most part, Reassessing an injury is quite similar to resting and recovering after an injury.

Reassessment doesn't just happen once. It happens daily or even several times a day in the first days and weeks following a concussion. Some of the steps involved in reassessing may include:

- Asking yourself some hard questions and making good observations
- Neuropsychological testing
- Consulting the Symptom Checklist

- Assessing your balance/vestibular function
- Assessing your coordination

## Ask the Difficult Questions when Reassessing

Think about these ways to Reassess yourself once you feel better:

- Evaluate how you feel when you watch TV (or text, read off a screen, etc.)
- Evaluate how you feel when you take a short jog around the neighborhood or track
- See what your health care provider says about your progress
- Determine what your school or team requires in terms of Rest before engaging in a return to activities/play protocol
- Find out what an honest self-assessment of the Symptom Checklist (in the appendix of this book) reveals
- Explore what it feels like to do a crossword puzzle, math problem, or read a story and recall details
- See whether you can stay focused on a movie
- Evaluate whether you can listen in class, take notes, and comprehend the material without getting a headache
- Determine whether you can concentrate at work without feeling fuzzy or dizzy

- Explore whether you can be productive without spending the rest of your day in bed with a headache
- Evaluate your score on a simple neuropsychological screening test, such as the ImPACT test. (No matter how you feel, these scores may reveal that your brain is not yet *objectively* ready to resume normal activities)
- Check whether you have unexplained emotional outbursts

## What is Neuropsychological testing?

Many school districts, teams, leagues, and athletic clubs are performing baseline neuropsychological (NP) tests on their students and athletes. NP tests can be extensive, detailed, time-consuming, and administered by licensed and highly trained psychologists who are expert in nuanced interpretation. These tests tend to reveal a great deal of information about the patient. They are also expensive and not always easily accessed immediately after an injury.

Over the past several years a number of brief computerized neuropsychological tests have been developed. These tests are more readily available and accessible to large numbers of individuals, institutions, and schools. Many school districts, teams, leagues, and athletic clubs now perform online baseline neuropsychological tests on their students and athletes. A few of these NP tests include Cogstate, Headminder, and ImPACT.

One of the more common of these tests is ImPACT testing. ImPACT is a standardized online test that has been shown to be useful as an *adjunct* to a good clinical history, physical exam, and other evaluation that can *help to determine* if a concussion is likely to have occurred. The test was developed at the University of Pittsburgh and has been widely adapted by professional, college, public, private, and club teams throughout the United States and abroad. It can guide clinicians, coaches, and concussed individuals and families in determining when it is safe to return to regular activities, both physical and mental.

The test consists of a twenty-minute series of "game-like" operations that evaluate the following:

- Verbal memory
- Visual memory
- Visual motor speed
- Reaction time
- Impulse control

If a school or other organization uses these tests as a baseline, that means that athletes are tested prior to the start of a season (usually every two years) and those results are used as a basis of comparison should a head injury occur. The test is not an IQ test, and there are a number of factors that can affect the baseline scores. These include:

- history of attention deficit disorder
- learning disabilities
- medications
- lack of sleep
- effort put into the test
- previous concussions or brain injury
- gender
- age
- poor test-taking conditions
- recent exercise

Such tests are not black-and-white. They require interpretation. The developers of the ImPACT test at the University of Pittsburgh provide a class and continuing education courses that certify clinicians and athletic trainers in the interpretation of the test.

It should also be noted that the test is a screening tool and is only one factor in determining whether a person is ready to start challenging his or her brain following an injury. The ImPACT developers (www.Impacttest.com) themselves describe the test this way:

What ImPact IS and Isn't:

- IS a clinically useful and reliable/valid concussion management program
- IS a tool to help determine recovery from injury

- IS a <u>tool</u> to help determine return to play
- IS a <u>tool</u> to help manage concussion (e.g. return to exertion, return to academics)
- IS a <u>tool</u> to help communicate post-concussion status to coaches, parents, clinicians

- IS NOT a substitute for medical evaluation/ treatment
- IS NOT a stand-alone assessment program
- IS NOT effective if clinician is naïve to specifics and complexities of data

Even skilled neuropsychologists who regularly use sensitive and validated instruments such as this in their professional lives often ponder the meaning of shifts in numbers on particular tests following a concussion.

I often tell my patients that their symptoms will always trump the ImPACT test. In other words, if someone were to score nearly as well or even better than their personal baseline a week after a concussion, but was still experiencing headaches with exertion of any kind, he or she would still be required to rest for some period of time before an increase in physical and mental exertion would be recommended.

HOW TO USE IMPACT TESTING (or other NP testing) IF YOU HAVE BEEN BASELINE TESTED:

If you are in a school or other athletic program that uses ImPACT testing as part of its concussion management program, you will probably be tested at least once following your concussion and this information will be used in conjunction with your health care provider's assessment of your readiness to return to activities. Different providers and authorities will have different responsibilities as to the final say regarding your return. In many schools, the district physician has the final word.

But remember, if you think you are not ready to go back, even if you are cleared, the final say sits with YOU. It is all in YOUR head.

If school is closed or you otherwise do not have access to your baseline test, or if you never had a baseline test, it is possible to have an ImPACT test following a concussion with results that can still be useful.

There are standards and norms in the database where ImPACT was developed against which your post-injury testing can be compared. An experienced ImPACT interpreter will know how to use your test *in conjunction with a number of other* factors to help guide your recovery plan.

**Are there other ways you can actually Reassess yourself at home?**

The short answer is Yes. But it is a qualified yes. Of course it is impossible to be completely objective about your own results. On the other hand, as we have discussed previously, it is important to gauge your own progress, or lack of it, and not push too hard. In almost all situations, a final clearance from a health care provider is a good idea, even if not mandatory.

HOW DO YOU SELF-ADMINISTER A SYMPTOM CHECK LIST?

If you do not have access to either baseline or post-injury testing, it is still possible to use other somewhat objective methods to assess your recovery. The symptom checklist is one such method.

A version of the symptom checklist developed by the National Association of Athletic Trainers and used by many clinicians, the ImPACT test, which is mentioned above and is recommended by the American Academy of Pediatrics, appears in the appendix of this book.

It was suggested earlier that you have someone read the list to you in the first 24 hours after the injury. This is important since you are not supposed to be reading or doing any "brain work" during this vital period.

If you are feeling better, it is OK to administer the test every 48 hours or so. If you are not seeing a health care provider who administers something similar or asks you the relevant questions, it is okay to administer the test to yourself. If you are seeing a health care provider, copy the form and take it along to show your progress (or lack of it). Keep in mind:

- Be honest
- Record your symptoms from the last 24 hours only
- Have someone read the list and score it for you if you have trouble doing it on your own

**And how do I assess balance or vestibular function?**

"Vestibular" refers to the delicate system in the inner ear that connects to the brain and is responsible for balance and a sense of where the body is in space.

Vestibular function is very sensitive to concussion injury and testing this function is a valuable way to determine whether the brain has recuperated fully from injury. It stands to reason that most athletes rely on their balance, at one point or another, to perform optimally. I have often tested athletes who think they are ready to return to sports, only to be stunned by how "off" their sense of balance is when they are put through this test. But everyone, whether an athlete or not, needs a sense of balance to perform daily activities safely.

There are high-tech balance assessment systems that are used in academic centers and in studies of concussion injury and recovery. But there is another "low-tech" test, called the Balance Error Scoring System, or BESS, that was first developed at the University of North Carolina at Chapel Hill. Athletic trainers and physicians as well as physical therapists have adopted this and it is part of the Sports Concussion and Assessment Tool 2 (or SCAT2) widely used by schools, leagues, and sports organizations around the country, and even in the Olympics, as part of the overall assessment of readiness to return to activity.

It is possible to do a mini-version of this test at home. *But you should not do this alone.*

Here are the directions to one component of the BESS. Have your partner read this to you:

"The first stance is standing with your feet together with your hands on your hips and with your eyes closed. You should try to maintain stability in that position for 20 seconds. I will be counting the number of times you move out of this position. I will start timing when you are set and have closed your eyes."

The other two parts of the BESS test are in the Appendix to the book. If you can easily do the one above, then you might want to try the other two. One test involves standing with feet in a tandem position for 20 seconds and the other involves standing on one leg for 20 seconds.

You might get better with practice but it's not a good idea to practice this *at all* if doing so gives you a headache or you are not otherwise ready to return to activities for any of the other reasons discussed in this chapter.

**And how about the test of coordination?**

This test also requires a partner but does not incur any risk of falling and is actually likely to induce the giggles. It's called the "Finger-to-nose" test. Not what you are thinking! Have your partner simply watch you while you sit in a chair and with an outstretched arm (first test the right; then the left) you simply move as quickly as possible from a fully extended arm to touching the tip of your nose to the extended arm five successive times. The goal is to do this accurately 5 times in less than 4 seconds.

*When should you Return to Activities and Play? ONCE you feel you are functioning well; you are down to a symptom score below 5 or 6; your balance score is back to normal; and your coordination is up to speed. But beware. This is supposed to be a gradual process.*

## What is a general "Return to Play Plan of Action" for most people?

Please note that this plan applies to athletes as well as to individuals who are average folks who walk ten blocks to work, like to get out to play tennis once or twice a week, take a walk around the neighborhood, go dancing on weekends, or even just need to climb a few flights of stairs on a daily basis.

In general, the concept is:

- to follow a step-wise progression of increasing activity that slowly increases the heart rate (and therefore the stress on the brain and its energy demands)
- to slow the progress from one stage to the next if symptoms (anything from the checklist, but most commonly fatigue and headache) occur when you push to the next level
- 24 hours or longer should elapse between each stage, as long as there are no symptoms

For example:

1.  Rest until symptom-free (physical and mental rest) THIS, OF COURSE, IS THE POINT OF THIS WHOLE BOOK
2.  Light aerobic exercise (stationary bike, a walk around the block, one flight of stairs, walk the dog for five minutes)
3.  A sport-specific exercise (a short jog, a slow skate around the rink, a jog across the field, a quick jog around the court, a quick easy tennis game)
4.  Non-contact training drills (light resistance training may begin)
5.  Full contact training should only start after medical clearance
6.  Game play and full competition

In general, the rule to follow is that if symptoms return, the brain is not healed.

You need to go back.

This is what we mean by Reassess.

Rethink it.

You probably need more Rest.

Reassess. Rest.

Reassess again.

# Chapter Ten:
## When It Might Take Longer to Get Better

Most concussion experts agree that there are several factors that are likely to modify the recovery trajectory for a given individual following a head injury.

Listen to some of our eyewitness accounts:

> *"I still experience sensitivity to light and I experience difficulty recalling recent conversations and daily occurrences (i.e. phone conversations, movies that I've seen, etc.)"*
> MN, age 17, female, two years after injury

> *"My short-term memory is awful, could be from the concussion or just genetics, my Dad has trouble remembering things sometimes as well. I am convinced concussions have affected my personality, I think I am a little moodier because of them. I notice I occasionally stumble over pronouncing some of my words, some days are worse than others."*
> NN, age 31, male, suffered at least 10 concussions

*"I didn't return to the field for about 2 months. I had a concussion back in college and knew I needed to wait to give my brain time to heal. I didn't feel normal for probably 3 weeks. "*
RD, age 26, male, rugby player

*"...how little the doctors seem to know about how long each individual's symptoms will last!! This kind of surprised me and I saw a top neurologist in the city!"*
OR, 56, female, tripped on sidewalk

**What does this mean?**

We have said previously that the recovery process is very individual and is often described as a moving target. However, experienced clinicians have noted that there are certain categories of people who clearly have a more difficult time fully recuperating from a concussion.

Any clinician who sees a patient following a head injury should inquire about any history of these modifying factors:

- Number of symptoms (i.e. from the Symptom Checklist)
- Duration of symptoms lasting more than ten days
- Severity of symptoms
- Loss of consciousness for more than one minute
- Amnesia (especially for events prior to the injury)

- Convulsions
- A history of previous concussions (exact numbers not known or studied)
- Recent concussion (unclear how recent is "too" recent with risks of Second Impact Syndrome, post concussion syndrome or simply a prolonged recovery)
- Change in threshold: meaning that a concussion has occurred with a seemingly lesser degree of impact or that recovery has been slower with successive hits
- Age: children and adolescents are at increased risk; at least until age 18 and possibly older as the brain continues growing until about age 25
- Other issues: migraine headache history; depression or other mental illness; ADHD; ADD; learning disabilities; sleep disorders
- Medication: psychoactive drugs; anticoagulants (blood thinners)
- Behavior: dangerous style of play
- Gender: Females are thought to be at increased risk due to their less developed neck muscles. It is unclear if there are other factors that may make females more vulnerable to concussion

If a person has one or more of the modifying factors, it *may* mean that recovery could take longer than average. It may also mean that he or she would be best managed by a team of expert clinicians who are experienced in managing concussion. Not every pediatrician, neurologist, or doctor who does ImPACT testing knows how to manage concussions. So ask questions. Ask, when you make the initial phone call whether he or she has managed post concussion syndrome. Don't waste your time or theirs!

As time goes on and recovery is slow or frustrating, **secondary symptoms** (such as depression and anxiety) will often emerge. Having a supportive team that knows how to manage these symptoms can make a big difference in planning for the patient's school or work and his or her mental, social, and physical well-being. That team may involve the following members:

- Social worker
- Guidance counselor
- Psychologist
- Psychiatrist
- Neurologist
- Neuropsychologist
- Educational psychologist
- Physical therapist
- Acupuncturist
- Massage therapist

Sometimes medication may be prescribed for any of the following complications of concussion. It would be uncommon to prescribe medications before a few weeks of natural, simple rest and recovery have elapsed. But more work will undoubtedly be done in the field of medicating concussion symptoms as more concussions are recognized.

Symptoms that may require treatment with prescription medications include:

- Sleep disturbances
- Migraine headaches
- Severe concussion headaches
- Foggy thinking
- Difficulty concentrating
- Depression

In general, if a patient requires prescription medications following a head injury (and did not require them before), he or she should remain on limited physical activity, low concussive risk activities, and cognitive restrictions (meaning some school adjustments), if necessary. Patients like these will usually require a more advanced neuropsychological assessment by someone who is familiar with head injury and educational issues, particularly if school modifications are a concern.

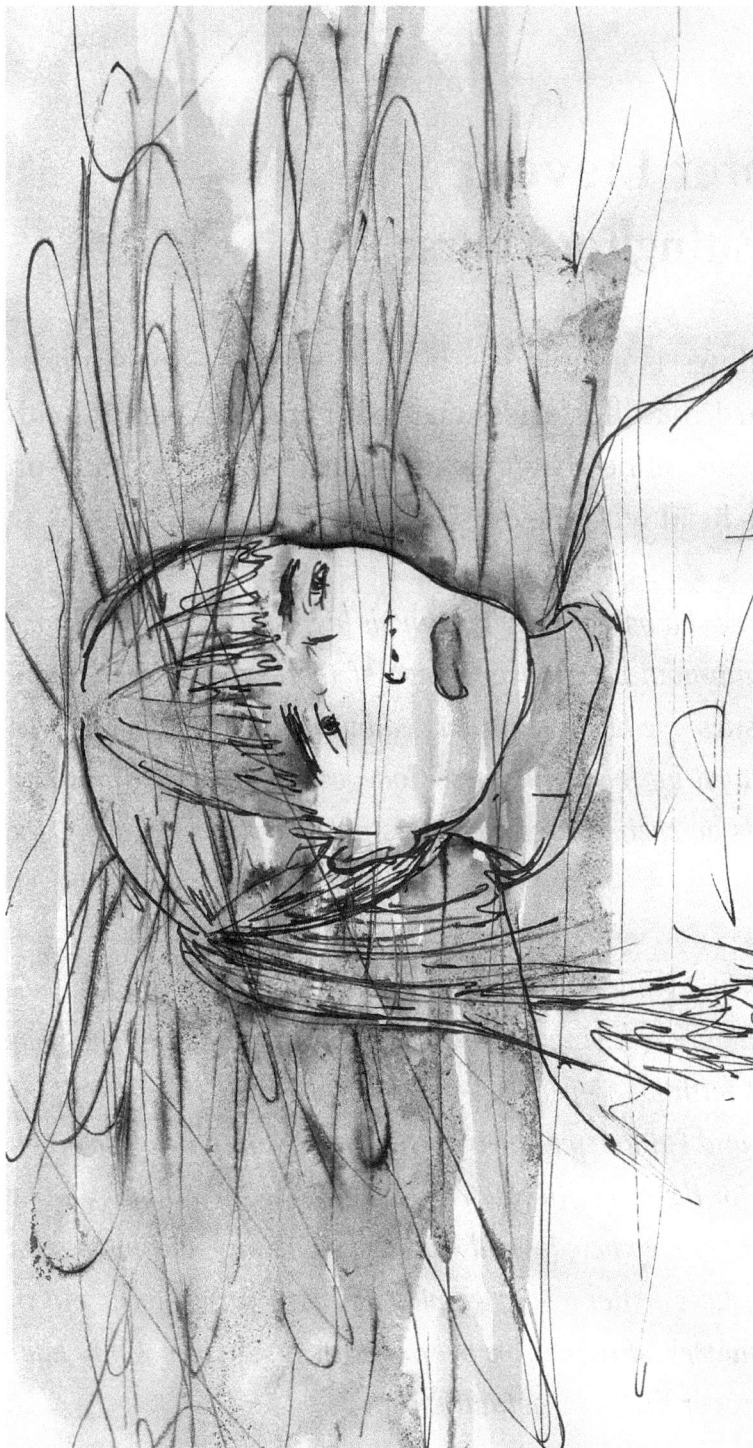

" ….a potent feeling of pain and anxiety"

# Chapter Eleven:
## Advocating for Yourself

What follows is a fable based on a composite of stories I have heard that illustrates what happens to a person with a concussion as he struggles to reconcile what is going on inside his head with the outside world.

*Xavier is the star basketball player in his high school. His handsome face has appeared on the front page of the local newspaper and local websites. He has been promoted by the Lions Club and been congratulated by local charities. Colleges have scouted him and he depends on their courtship for his plan to play D1 ball in the future.*

*In last night's game Xavier went up for a shot, was blocked and lost his balance, causing him to fall backwards, hitting the floor hard, first with his upper back and then the back of his head. He saw stars and felt dizzy as he tried to get up. Coach had him sit on the bench for the rest of the quarter. His head was pounding but he did not let on. He knew he had had his "bell rung" but he refused to say anything. After a botched play, he asked to be subbed out in the final quarter, sure that the team lost because of him. Only later did he discover that they actually won.*

*Later that evening, after a dinner his mom left for him on the stove before she left for her night shift at the hospital, he headed for a shower. As he downed three Advil, he listened to the voicemail on the home phone left by Coach calling to check on him.*

*He did not return the call but instead headed to bed, barely able to stay awake a minute longer, and fell asleep. He couldn't even take time to worry that the next day his stepfather was coming to town to watch him play against the big rival, Central High. His dad had not seen him play since Xavier grew three inches last year and was named MVP.*

ↁ

By now, if you've read any part of this book, you know that Xavier has had a concussion.

We **Recognize** the initial symptoms of seeing stars, confusion, and an immediate headache. We see that Xavier did not **Respond** quite the way he should have at first; neither did his coach. Xavier continued to play instead of being benched immediately after a blow that left him with a headache and feeling stunned and confused.

Only Xavier understood at that moment that something dangerous had happened. *It was all in his head at that moment.* It was up to him to make the call. Fortunately, finally asking to be subbed out was the wisest thing he did. And fortunately, the coach tried to make contact with him at home later that evening. But we feel dismayed and nervous that Xavier was left alone without any supervision after his injury. In spite of all this, Xavier knew that **Rest** is what he needed.

☙

*The next morning, Xavier was still in bed when his mom came home from work. When he told her what happened and that he was still feeling dizzy and had a headache, she immediately suspected a concussion and told him he would be missing not only school but also the big game that night.*

*Xavier felt too lousy to fight back. His mom decided to take him to the doctor for an evaluation and an ImPACT test, which showed a marked change from his baseline test that had been done at school during the pre-season.*

## HOW DO I TALK TO MY DOCTOR?

It is important to accurately report your symptoms to your doctor. Many physicians are aware of new policies and thinking about concussion but some still are not.

Tell the story as it happened. If a family member was with you or heard the story from witnesses, have them come along and tell the story with you.

Report **all** of your symptoms. They will generally fall into four categories, similar to the Symptom Checklist in the Appendix.

**Physical symptoms:**
Visual problems
Balance issues
Sensitivity to light
Sensitivity to sound
Nausea
Headaches (describe the kind and location of headache)
Dizziness

**"Cognitive" symptoms (of the mind):**
Memory issues
Attention problems
Problems focusing
Fatigue
Slow thinking
Feeling "foggy"

**Emotional disruption:**
Sadness
Irritability
Nervousness
Crankiness

**Sleep instability:**

Difficulty getting to sleep

Difficulty staying awake

What seems like an excessive need for sleep

*The doctor told Xavier that he had a concussion, just as he and his mother had both suspected. His "prescription" for Xavier, which he wrote out on one of his regular prescription pads, was for "bed rest."*

*"You will not be able to play for the next seven to ten days, Xavier. I don't want you to do any exercise that will increase your heart rate more than 20 points over baseline. You are going to be bored and probably grumpy. But otherwise you will have a terrible headache and you will not heal quickly from this concussion."*

*Immediately Xavier started to protest. The first thing he thought about but didn't say out loud was, "What about my dad?" What he did say was: "How am I going to tell my coach? He's expecting me to play in the big game on Friday against Central!"*

*The doctor told him that if the coach understands that he has had a concussion, the coach will also understand that it is his responsibility not to play Xavier until he has had a chance to heal. The doctor also explained that he would have to see him and evaluate another ImPACT test in a few more days to chart his recovery. He explained that the ImPACT test could be done at school, if Xavier felt like going to school, but only if he did not feel worse being in the hustle and bustle of the high school hallways.*

*The doctor reminded Xavier that the school's policy on concussions was very clear about not playing and therefore there was no room for discussion.*

*"You don't need to feel guilty about this, buddy. It's not your fault. It goes with the territory of being a Big Man on a great team. Would you like me to speak to Coach?"*

*"No," said Xavier, "I think I can handle this one. One of my buddies had a similar thing in football last fall. I think Coach knows. I actually think he suspected something was wrong." Xavier remembered the phone call the night before but didn't want his mom to know he had been too sick to pick up. She would have wanted to leave work to take care of him.*

## HOW DO I TALK TO MY PARENTS?

*Xavier left the doctor's office with his mom and felt exhausted from the experience, which is common after a concussion. After all, all those questions and thinking is "brain work" and can give a person with a concussion a headache. But the most difficult thing still lay ahead of him. How was he going to tell his dad?*

*At best, Xavier's relationship with his dad could be described as rocky, but he had been banking on this one opportunity to show his success at basketball and his success as a person in his school.*

*It was really something he had been looking forward to and it was not easy to give up. Furthermore, he was pretty sure his father would interpret this as Xavier's fault in some way, or call him a "wuss," or see him as weak (his father hadn't yet seen the extra three inches Xavier had grown) and he was coming all this way especially for the big game. Xavier was quite sure Dad would say, "Come on, I used to just get back on the field when I had my bell rung all the time. We all did."*

These are the types of dialogues people, and especially athletes, have with themselves all the time. But times have changed and sometimes patients with concussions will find themselves in the position of having to advocate for themselves and educate those around them about what it means to have a concussion and why they require the Rest and adjustments that they do. These are the words of a middle-schooler and former patient of mine, ML, age 14, who had to sit out his big hockey game because of a concussion:

> *"The white jerseys file out of the room and onto the ice. I stay on the bench, thinking about our loss to S last night. I wish I had been able to play, but instead I was useless cheerleader on the sideline. I should hate hockey for all that it's done to me, but I can't wait to lace up next fall."*

Xavier needs only to show his dad the policies of his school or the headlines in the news on a nearly weekly — if not daily — basis, or download this book for his dad so that he will understand that those who care about Xavier and others with head injuries are doing the right thing by having him miss a game or a week, but sparing perhaps his whole life, both as an athlete and as a student.

## HOW DO I TALK TO MY SCHOOL/WORKPLACE?

*At this point Xavier's Mom asked the doctor what they should do about school and homework, midterms, the SATs in two weeks, and the job interview Xavier had scheduled for an internship during his upcoming spring break.*

*The doctor advised them to take things a day at a time. Most concussions are better in one to three weeks.(Xavier's eyes rolled when he heard this. Rolling his eyes instantly increased his headache, by the way.) The doctor reminded Xavier and his mother that in the meantime it was the school's obligation to re-schedule tests, shorten class time, excuse absences, cut back on homework, adjust due dates for papers, and allow for extra time, if necessary. Much of these adjustments are no different than those that would be granted for a person who had an appendectomy or a bad case of mononucleosis.*

*The doctor gave them some common sense advice as well. Now would not be a good time to go on an interview, but in two weeks Xavier might be well enough to make that the focus of his day, or even be completely healed by then. The day after an injury it is impossible to predict just how long recovery will take. Rest is the keystone of recovery, the doctor reminded them.*

ΩΩ ΩΩ ΩΩ ΩΩ

As we have discussed and demonstrated, the effects of a concussion are not just physical. In fact, most people describe the mental and emotional effects as being the most debilitating. Furthermore, not all concussions occur in athletes but many patients are students and almost all patients have responsibilities either at school or work.

The academic environment can be extremely helpful in making adjustments to learning during the recovery period. Colleges may have offices of disability services and they are sometimes the best advocate a college student may have when she is away from home. These offices are frequently thought of as places that serve students with chronic problems but they also can be strong advocates and coaches for students who have temporary disabling conditions such as post concussion syndrome.

The suggestions in the remainder of this chapter are taken from Karen McAvoy's 2012 article "Return to Learning: Going Back to School Following a Concussion" published in Communiqué, the online publication of the National Association of School Psychologists.

In order to help organize one's thoughts on "How can I get the help I need?" it is useful to organize the academic problems into three areas of cognitive, or brain, functioning:

- Mental fatigue
- Slowed Processing
- Difficulty with new learning

**Mental Fatigue**:

As we discovered in Chapter 6 during recovery from a concussion the primary disturbance is an energy deficit in the brain. This results in *exhaustion* when the brain is pushed beyond its reserves. Adjustments in the daily schedule can include the following, but creative suggestions, often coming from the patient/student/athlete himself are often the most successful:

- Shorter days, if necessary. Since most concussed individuals experience increased headache as the day goes on, it would be best to start the day at the normal time and come home early. Although many a teenager would prefer to go in at 11 and stay until three, this is not really what the brain needs. Once recovery is underway, experts suggest increasing the time at school as quickly as possible even if it means more academic adjustments so that the student does not fall behind socially and developmentally.

- Provide 15-20 minute rest periods throughout the day. A school nurse or guidance counselor may need to help determine the best place or places for the student to take breaks.

- Some suggest taking "strategic" rest periods. This means they are *scheduled in.* It is better not to wait until a headache or sense of exhaustion have begun.

- Adjustment in the amount of in-class work and homework. Options will vary by class type, teacher and student symptoms. A student may be able to manage 10 math problems but not 20. A student may be able to attend a class but not produce a paper. A student may not be able to watch a PowerPoint presentation due to sensitivity to light but may be able to listen to an audio version if that is possible. Creativity and compassion will be in order.

- A student may need to be excused from assemblies, concerts, games, or other events or areas of school where light, noise and crowds provoke a headache.

- Teachers and administrators need to be aware that emotional factors may be part of the symptom complex and students may be experiencing irritability and unstable emotions.

## Slowed Processing

If a student is experiencing a slowing in processing speed, he will still be able to learn and do work but usually at a much slower pace. These are McAvoy's suggested adjustments:

- Cut back on the work given in class and for homework. Quality of work is more important than quantity. An overload can easily provoke a headache or other symptoms and a relapse in a person recovering from concussion.
- Extra time should be given for tests and projects. Some would argue that testing during the recovery period is unfair all together.
- Use technology to make all tasks, from note taking to reviewing lectures more stress free.
- Enlist helpers and assistants where appropriate.
- Adjust due dates or cancel projects all together.

## Difficulty with new learning

Students who are recovering from concussion will have trouble retaining new material in memory but will also have difficulty with new concepts. So the very basis of learning is impaired and expectations need to be altered. As a result students, parents and teachers may benefit from these simple suggestions:

- Teachers may need to explicitly point out the most important points in their lesson plan
- Older students may need to explicitly ask to be given a list of the salient points of a lecture
- Again, it may not be fair to base a semester grade test or judge an important project at this time due to an impairment in learning.
- Focus should be on understanding rather than on rote memorization or detail. Perhaps a discussion rather than a test would help to evaluate the student's status and can serve the dual purpose of showing support.
- Many concussed students will need to have their workload cut back not just postponed. It may be impossible to catch up later.

The rules of the games are changing and the ways in which we all respond to our sons, daughters, students, players, and friends are also evolving. And that is how we will prevent more head injuries, and more severe head injuries, in the future. Read on for more discussion about ways to prevent concussions in yourself and others.

In summary, as with other aspects of concussion management, much of it depends on the injured person him or herself. He or she needs to step up and recognize, respond and reassess the ever fluid and ongoing situation whether it is in the first minutes, hours and days following the injury or in the ensuing weeks. Only you will know whether that French test was really your best effort or if something is still not working right inside your head.

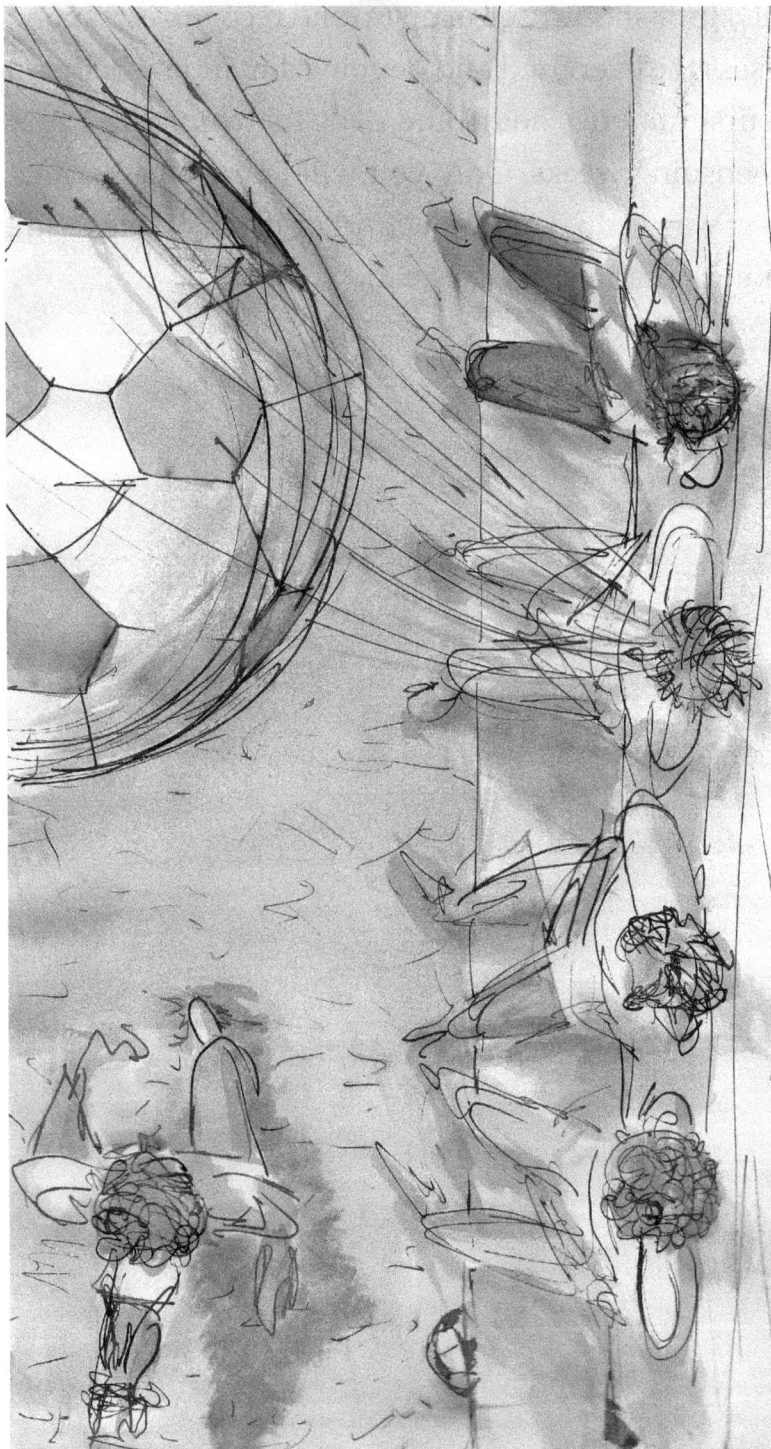

"they said it would be safe to go to the game but I got hit by a stray ball just watching"

# Chapter Twelve:
## How Can This Be Prevented?

**So how can we prevent concussions from happening?**

It is probably safe to say that we will never be able to prevent all concussions. Life happens. People trip and fall. We engage in contact sports. Car accidents will happen.

But the elderly should be prevented from falling out of bed. Football players need not lead with their heads; children can wear helmets when riding bikes; and people can drive sober.

In addition, it should be clear from reading and understanding the Four Rs (Recognize, Respond, Rest, and Reassess) in this book that by correctly responding to a concussion we can actually help prevent the next one from happening, which we discussed at some length in Chapter Two: The Four Rs and the Four Ds.

Only a few months ago I presented a brief talk to several hundred parents, athletes, and coaches from my local high school's fall sports teams. I addressed our school's comprehensive and conservative concussion policy. The final slide I showed was a cartoon by Hafeez that had just appeared in the *New Yorker* magazine, of a football huddle where the coach is saying to his players, "Now promise me you will all be very careful." I suggested that because of what we now know about concussions, there may actually have to be some changes in the rules of the game.

As I returned to my seat a rather intense father leaned over to me and said, "Gee, Doc, what are you going to do? Stop the kids from tackling? I played rough my whole life." I quietly suggested that we would just have to see what would happen.

The very next morning, Pop Warner, a national athletic league for almost half a million kids ages 5 to 16, announced a change in the rules of football practice.

The following rules were announced in June 2012 on the Pop Warner website (www.PopWarner.com) in direct response to growing concerns about concussions in young players:

**The New Rules Are as Follows:**
- No full speed head-on blocking or tackling drills in which the players line up more than 3 yards apart are permitted. (Having two linemen in stances immediately across the line of scrimmage from each other and having full-speed drills where the players approach each other at an angle, but not straight

ahead in to each other are both permitted.) **<u>However,
there should be no intentional head-to-head contact!</u>**

- The amount of contact at each practice will be reduced
  to a maximum of 1/3 of practice time (either 40
  minutes total of each practice or 1/3 of total weekly
  practice time). In this context, "contact" means any
  drill or scrimmage in which drills; down line vs. down
  line full-speed drills; and scrimmages.

In addition to these changes, Pop Warner also announced
that there would no longer be butt blocking, chop blocking,
face tackling or spearing techniques permitted in the game
of football.

**What else can we do to prevent concussions?**

In 2010, the NFL (www.nfl.com) announced a rule change to
address the issue of head injury in players. "The reworded
rules prohibit a player from launching himself off the ground
and using his helmet to strike a player in a defenseless
posture in the head or neck. The old rule only applied to
receivers getting hit, but now it will apply to everyone."

Pop Warner and the NFL have weighed in with their
recommendations on changing the established rules of the
game, but we have to ask what else might be done to help
prevent head injury.

## Does equipment matter?

There is a great deal of confusion, debate, and study about whether helmets, mouth guards, and other equipment or even training can prevent concussion. Most objective experts at this point will say "not really."

Helmets have a role to play in preventing cuts and bruises and probably in preventing skull fractures but seem to have a limited role in actually preventing concussion. Some even argue that helmets give a false sense of security, that athletes play harder, and even lead with their heads under the false assumption that their skulls are protected by the head gear. In a 2009 review of the scientific literature on the subject in the *British Journal of Sports Medicine*, it was found that most studies have significant limitations in evaluating the efficacy of helmets in reducing the risk of concussion. Among these limitations is the fact that the sponsors of the studies are often the helmet manufacturers themselves. Clearly, this is an area where more work is required.

In the meantime, concussion prevention *for the most part* depends on "playing nice," playing elegantly, and on enforcing the rules. Finally, concussion prevention will also depend on following proper management once a head injury has occurred.

**However, there are a few other pieces of advice that most experts recommend to parents and community leaders:**

- Basic protective gear should be properly fitted and appropriate to the activity or sport. This includes protective eye, mouth, and shin guards; padding, and helmets.
- If possible, have your child undergo a baseline neuropsychological test (such as ImPACT, if it is available at your school). You may be able to find baseline testing outside of school if it is not available through school-based team sports.
- Let your child know that sportsmanlike conduct is expected as part of your family's values. Unsportsmanlike conduct often leads to injury.
- If your child has ADD or ADHD, be sure he or she is properly medicated for games, even if after school, when kids often think they don't "need" medication. Remember: inattentive or impulsive play can contribute to injury.
- Be sure coaches and trainers are aware of the new rules, recommendations, and laws about head injury.
- Educate yourself about head injury. Go to cdc.gov for your own tutorial. Invite other parents to do the same. Share this book with others for some great stories and anecdotes.
- FINALLY, teach children the signs of concussion, encourage them, and *give them permission* to withdraw

from an activity if they think they have sustained an
injury.

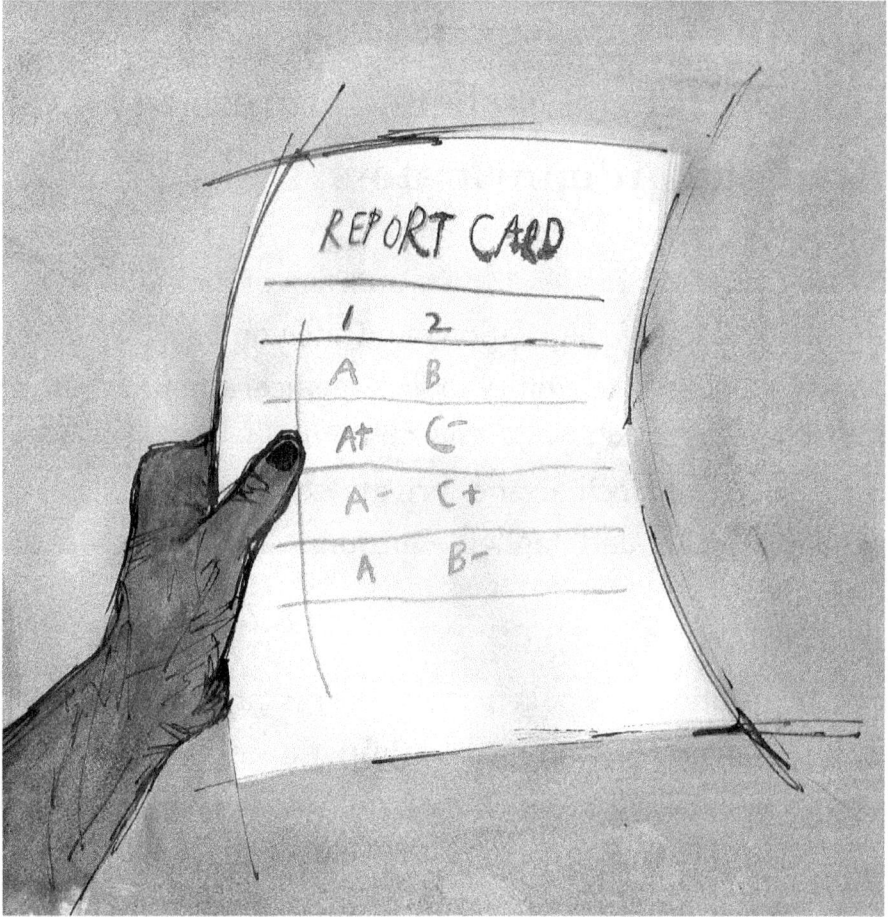

"...she started having trouble concentrating and kept insisting she had ADD."

# Chapter Thirteen:
## For Doctors, Teachers, Professors, and Academic Administrators

By August of 2012 at least three-quarters of the states in the country had passed legislation requiring youths who sustain a sports-related brain injury to seek medical attention before returning to activities within the public school system. Increasingly, parochial and private schools are adopting similar policies and higher education should not be far behind.

This legislation has taken many forms and has recently included an understanding of the importance of the cognitive as well as the physical recovery required after a head injury. Known as RTL or Return to Learning, this phase of recovery may impact more people in the academic community and for a longer period of time than RTP or Return to Play. As we have previously discussed in this book, there can be very subtle signs of trouble during the recovery period; signs that may only be apparent to the concussed individual.

The New York State Guidelines issued in June 2012 outline specific roles for different members of the community including doctors, school nurses, teachers, administrators, and pupil personnel service staff. This chapter will build on those guidelines and serve as a starting point for some of these professionals who may be mandated to help concussed students.

This chapter does not discuss the roles of coaches, certified athletic trainers, athletic directors, school health personnel, and school district physicians. These critical professionals whose training and licensure often involves specific education about concussion will work as a team under the new guidelines to develop and implement clinical policies and act as front line reporters as well as critical coordinators with all of the other members of this very large and important team.

**What are the Responsibilities of the School Administrator/ Pupil Personnel Services Staff (PPS) Regarding Concussions in Students?**

- Organize a team of personnel to create a concussion management team

- Create a concussion management policy, including privacy/permission forms, RTP forms, and communication forms between athletic staff, health staff, guidance, and administrative staff

- Assign one person to be a communicator in the district or community about concussion policy

- Develop educational programs for students, staff, teachers, coaches, athletic trainers, guidance and psychology staff

- Develop chains of communication between all of the departments that need to know if a child/student has had a concussion, whether the injury occurred in school or out

- Ensure that teachers/professors know "what to look for" and when to refer for extra guidance

- Ensure that all legal procedures (FERPA-Family Educational Rights and Privacy Act) are followed in communicating between the school and private providers

- Encourage parents (in the case of a minor) to share outside medical and psychological evaluation with the appropriate school personnel for optimal cooperation

Most administrators in the public sector quake at the thought of the budgetary implications of the tremendous potential for increase in accommodations, 504 plans, extra help, increased technology, and other services that may be required by students who have a prolonged illness or disability.

It should be understood that most concussed students, *if managed correctly from the outset with the Four Rs laid out in detail in this book,* will do well and require no more special instruction or care than the average student with mononucleosis, pneumonia, or a bad case of the flu. A small percentage of students will go on to have prolonged post concussion syndrome and will need special adjustments in their curriculum or accommodations. A clear understanding of these issues from the outset on the part of all members of the academic community will head off complications at the pass.

## What Are the Responsibilities of the Community Doctor?

- All medical doctors seeing children, young adults, and athletes who may have had a head injury should have taken continuing medical education credits in concussion management. They can do this independently through the CDC's website (www.cdc.gov).

- If clinicians do not feel competent or up to date in making decisions according to current thinking, they should refer patients out until they are up to speed.

- If clinicians are not familiar with ImPACT or other neuropsychological testing and are presented with such a test as part of the evaluation of a concussed patient, they should seek advice from someone who is certified in interpretation or refer the patient on.

- All schools will require a definite statement and assessment from a doctor as to whether a student has sustained a "concussion." Although the school might then request orders as to restrictions and monitoring, many schools will now have, as part of their own concussion management protocol, an established restriction on student participation in PE, gym, sports, competition, etc., that overrides your own orders.

- Many schools will have their own Return to Play protocol. If you wish to provide your own, you can find it at the SCAT2 app that is downloadable for free on your computer or mobile phone.

- Be available to communicate with the school nurse, athletic trainer, medical director, guidance counselor, or other school personnel. It pays to listen to their judgment and observations; they know the student in his or her everyday context.

- Be conservative. Do not bow to pressure to allow the patient to return to activities before a safe time period has elapsed. If in doubt, see the patient back in the office and do some simple tests (BESS, Symptom checklist, finger to nose, recall tests on SCAT2, ImPACT if available).

- The most important contribution you can make is to talk to your patient and the family and educate them about the dangers of returning to play or school too soon. Give them perspective on the inherent dangers of returning too quickly.

- When the time comes, you will need to provide written clearance, usually on a standard form provided by the student's school district.

- Do not make the mistake of returning the student to play or activity if he or she is not up to speed (or at least at baseline) academically. Academic and physical readiness should go hand in hand.

## What are the Responsibilities of the Teachers?

Once a student is back at school (and that could be the day after a concussion, in some cases) the teacher may be the adult spending the most time with the student and therefore in a position to observe and intervene if necessary. This is indeed an opportunity to help improve, and maybe even save, a student's life.

Teachers should be aware of the impact of concussion on the brain. The very subtle ways in which all of the brain functions can be affected have been discussed in earlier chapters in this book. To summarize, problems may arise in attention and concentration, speech and language, learning and memory, reasoning, planning, executive functioning, problem solving, and emotional and social dysfunction.

The appendix of this book lists some of the websites from the New York state guidelines that may be useful for teachers.

Encourage your district to organize workshops on concussion.

Collaborate with guidance, psychology and educational psychologists, including those in the district who are using and interpreting ImPACT tests to discuss results with you.

Discuss with a special education colleague a particular student you may be concerned about. Simple solutions may make a huge difference in just a few days.

Some other practical points that may help students as they make a gradual return to school and learning:

- Shorten the school day
- Give them breaks; e.g. twenty minutes of class time, twenty minutes of rest

- Allow extended time to complete tests
- Excuse them from tests altogether right after injury (And don't overload with too much makeup material: relapse may result)
- Copy your notes for them
- Give alternative assignments
- Allow peers to take notes
- Give verbal and non-verbal cues to help focus

❧

It should be noted that once doctors, teachers, and administrators are aware of the protean manifestations of concussion they will become much more astute observers, inquirers, and professionals. This will allow them to be more compassionate and effective in their work.

In times of economic hardship when there is little extra money in most budgets for fancy programs or expensive technology, a better set of eyes and ears and a well-honed sensitivity to the possibility that the presenting symptoms and behavior just might be due to concussion can be life-saving to the child or young adult and extremely gratifying to a stressed professional.

# About the Author

Ann Engelland is a pediatrician with over thirty years experience caring for children, teens, and young adults. Her specialty training and board certification is in adolescent medicine. After many years in private practice in Westchester County, New York, she now works in the public schools as the physician for two different districts and in the Barnard College student health service in New York City. In 2008, she directed the development and implementation of the concussion management policy for the Mamaroneck School District.

Her other credentials include her website and blog, www. AnnEngellandMD.com, where she comments on a spectrum of matters affecting the health and wellbeing of teens and young adults. Topics of discussion include safety, sexuality, infectious diseases, immunization practices, and current events affecting young people, families, and parents. Over the past two years raising awareness about head injury and concussion has been the subject of many of her posts.

Ann is the lucky mother of seven healthy children ages 19 to 31. Several of them now recognize that they sustained head injuries they would now call "concussions." It is partly because of their stories and those of Ann's patients that the Questionnaire and this book were born.

# Acknowledgments

This book could not have been written without the help of several key people and supporters. I would like to thank my daughter, Alice Taranto, for her creative work in illustrating the questionnaires; Jose Almaguer for his cover design; Alex Decicco for her dedication to research and knowledge; Stacey Vollman Warwick and Steven W. Booth for introducing me to the eBook world; my editor, Elizabeth Ridley for her eagle eye; all of the friends, friends of friends, patients, and friends of patients who responded to the Questionnaire with honesty and made it possible to truly illustrate this book; and finally to Jo, who supports me and walks with me everywhere.

# References

*Scholarly Journal Articles and Periodicals*

Barkhoudarian, G., Hovda, D. A., & Giza, C. C. (2011). The molecular pathophysiology of concussive brain injury. *Clinical Sports Medicine, 30*(1), 33-48.
Bey, T. & Ostick, B. (2009). Second impact syndrome. *Western Journal of Emergency Medicine, 10*(1), 6-10.

DeMatteo, C., Hanna, S., Mahone, W., Hollenberg, R., Scott, L., Law, M., Newman, A., Lin, C., & Xu, L. (2010). My child doesn't have a brain injury, he only has a concussion. *Pediatrics, 125*(2), 327-334.

Field, J. M., Hazinski, M. F., Sayre, M. R., Chameides, L., Schexnayder, M., Hemphill, M. F., et al (2010). 2010 American Heart Association guidelines for cardiopulmonary resuscitation and emergency cardiovascular care service. *Circulation, 122*(18).

Guskiewicz, K. M. (2003). Assessment of postural stability following sport-related concussion. *Current Sports Medicine*

*Reports, 2,* 24-30.

Halstead, M. E. & Walter, K. D. (2010). Clinical report-Sport-related concussion in children and adolescents. *Pediatrics, 126* (3), 597-615.

Lovell, M. R., Collins, M.W., Iverson, G.L., Johnston, K.M., & Bradley, J.P. (2004). Grade 1 or "Ding" concussions in high school athletes. *The American Journal of Sports Medicine, 32(47).*

McAvoy, K. (2012). Return to learning: Going back to school following a concussion. *Communiqué, 40* (6). Retrieved from http://www.nasponline.org/publications/cq/40/6/return-to-learning.aspx

McCrory, P., Meeuwisse, W., Johnston, K., Dvorak, J., Aubrey, M. Molloy, M., & Cantue, R. (2009). Consensus statement on concussion in sport: The 3rd international conference on concussion in sport held in Zurich, November 2008. *Journal of Athletic Training, 44(4),* 434-448.

Meeghan, W. P. & Bachur, R. G. (2009). Sport-related concussion. *Pediatrics, 123(1),* 114-123.

*Online Databases*

Centers for Disease Control and Prevention (2012). Concussion and mild TBI. Retrieved from: http://www. cdc.gov/concussion/

Centers for Disease Control and Prevention (2012). Heads up: Concussion in youth sports. Retrieved from: http:// www.cdc.gov/concussion/HeadsUp/youth.html

*Online News Articles*

McAvoy, K. (2011). REAP the benefits of good concussion management. Rocky Mountain Youth Sports Medicine Institute. Retrieved from http://www.brainline.org/ content/2011/06/reap-the-benefits-of-good-concussion-management_pageall.html

McCune, M. (2012, July 25). Women boxers choose perilous path. *WNYC*. Retrieved from: http://www.wnyc.org/ articles/wnyc-news-2/2012/jul/25/women-boxers-choose-perilous-path/

McGrath, B. (2011, January 31). Does football have a future: The N.F.L. and the concussion crisis. *The New Yorker*. Retrieved from: http://www.newyorker.com/ reporting/2011/01/31/110131fa_fact_mcgrath

O'Connor, A. (2012, May 10). Concussions may be more severe in girls and young athletes. *The New York Times*. Retrieved from: http://well.blogs.nytimes.com/2012/05/10/concussions-may-be-more-severe-in-girls-and-young-athletes/

Schwarz, A. (2011, May 2). Duerson's brain trauma diagnosed. *The New York Times*. Retrieved from: http://www.nytimes.com/2011/05/03/sports/football/03duerson.html/

Schwarz, A. (2010, September 13). Suicide reveals signs of a disease seen in the N.F.L. *The New York Times*. Retrieved from: http://www.nytimes.com/2010/09/14/sports/14football.html?pagewanted=all

Sternberg, S. (2010, October 18). American Heart Association revises CPR guidelines. *USA Today*. Retrieved from: http://www.usatoday.com/yourlife/health/medical/2010-10-18-CPR18_ST_N.htm

*Podcasts and Interviews*

"Contact sport: Should heading be banned from youth soccer?" Narr. by Kate Snow. *Rock Center with Brian Williams*. NBC, 12 May 2012. *NBCNews*. Web. Retrieved 29 July 2012 from http://video.msnbc.msn.com/rock-center/47364254#47364254

"Dr. Sanjay Gupta reports: Big hits, broken dreams" Narr. by Sanjay Gupta. *CNN Presents.* CNN, 27 January 2012. Web. Retrieved 13 August 2012 from http://cnnpresents. blogs.cnn.com/2012/01/27/dr-sanjay-gupta-reports-big-hits-broken-dreams/

Dr. Mike Evans. (2011, December 16). *Concussions 101: A primer for kids and parents* [Video file]. Retrieved July 29, 2012, from http://www.youtube.com/watch?v=zCCD52Pty4A

Glicksman, B. (Interviewer) & Gupta, S. (Interviewee). (2012). A Q&A with Dr. Sanjay Gupta [Interview transcript]. Retrieved from SI.com: http://sportsillustrated.cnn. com/2012/writers/ben_glicksman/01/27/concussions. gupta.qanda/index.html

Gallegly, J. (2012, January 13). Balance Error Scoring System (BESS) demo. Retrieved August 15, 2012 from http://www. youtube.com/watch?v=xtJgv-D7IdU

Martin, M. (Interviewer) & Nowinski, C. (Interviewee). (2012). Is There A 'Concussion Crisis' In Sports? [Interview transcript]. Retrieved from National Public Radio Website: http://www.npr.org/2012/08/07/158361378/is-there-a-concussion-crisis-in-sports?sc=17&f=46

McCune, M. (Interviewer) & Chakour, V. (Interviewee). (2012). Go For It: Life Lessons From Girl Boxers [Interview audio file]. Retrieved from WNYC News: http://www.wnyc.org/articles/wnyc-news/2012/jul/12/go-for-it-life-lessons-girl-boxers/

Nowinski, C. (MSLawdotedu). (2012, April 14). Head games: The concussion crisis and the sports legacy institute. Retrieved July 29, 2012, from http://www.youtube.com/watch?v=YX_t5wLJQC0&feature=relmfu

Johnson, K. (Interviewee), McHale, L. (Interviewee), & Vietzke, H. (Interviewer). (2012). Head Trauma: The Wives Of Two Former NFL Players Discuss Their Husbands Issues [Interview audio file]. Retrieved from: http://www.youtube.com/watch?v=-8Kwfvy4vDI

*Books*

Meeghan, W. P. (2011). Kids, sports and concussion: A guide for coaches and parents. Santa Barbara, CA: The Praeger Series on Contemporary Health and Living.

*Government Documents*

The State Education Department. (2012). *Guidelines for concussion management in the school setting.* Albany, NY: Office of Student Support Services.

# Appendix

- Concussion Query (Questionnaire)
- Concussion Symptom Checklist
- Balance Error Scoring System (BESS)

# Concussion Query

A QUESTIONNAIRE FOR ANYONE WHO HAS EVER
SUSTAINED A HEAD INJURY

ANN L. ENGELLAND, MD

ADOLESCENT AND YOUNG ADULT MEDICINE

WWW.ANNENGELLANDMD.COM

THANKS

Thanks so much for helping me with this project. Time is of the essence. I hope to get this project out in the course of this summer. Your input and that of your friends and acquaintances is crucial.

I am interested in anything you have to say about your personal experiences with concussion or head injury. Your words and insight will contribute to a book that will help people better understand head injury and get the right treatment and care in order to recuperate and get back to normal, healthy activities as quickly as possible.

If you are certain you have had a concussion in the past, then you might find it relatively easy to answer these questions. You may *think* you have had a concussion but were never officially diagnosed. You are not alone. I also welcome *your* comments and recollections about such experiences.

Please answer in a different color or font and send this back to me as soon as you can. Your response will be your consent to use your words. You will be identified by initials and your age now and at the time of the injury.

Please forward this to any friends you have who may have sustained a head injury, in athletics or off the field. Many injuries occur from motor vehicle accidents, falls, and in countless other ways. I appreciate it and we can learn from all stories!

## QUESTIONNAIRE

Your initials? What is your DOB?

How many concussions do you think you have had? (If you have had multiple concussions, please indicate which one you are writing about.)

How old were you when you had the concussion/injury? What year was that?

Please write a paragraph about what happened to you. Whatever you recall is fine.

Did you think something serious was wrong? When did you realize that?

What were the symptoms you remember most?

How long do you think it took for you to get back to normal?

What kind of advice did you get about healing from your injury?

Did you alter your activities in any way after your concussion, either on your own or based on advice given?

How did the head injury affect your physical abilities?

How did the head injury affect your cognitive/mental abilities?

Were you affected emotionally by the injury? If so, how?

Anything else I should hear or know?

Thanks so much.

Date: _____

Ann Engelland, MD

## POST-CONCUSSION SYMPTOM SCALE

\* Please rate your symptoms over the last 24 hours

| SYMPTOMS | SEVERITY RATING | | | | | | |
|---|---|---|---|---|---|---|---|
| Balance Problems | 0 | 1 | 2 | 3 | 4 | 5 | 6 |
| Dizziness | 0 | 1 | 2 | 3 | 4 | 5 | 6 |
| Fatigue | 0 | 1 | 2 | 3 | 4 | 5 | 6 |
| Trouble falling asleep | 0 | 1 | 2 | 3 | 4 | 5 | 6 |
| Sleeping more than usual | 0 | 1 | 2 | 3 | 4 | 5 | 6 |
| Sleeping less than usual | 0 | 1 | 2 | 3 | 4 | 5 | 6 |
| Drowsiness | 0 | 1 | 2 | 3 | 4 | 5 | 6 |
| Sensitivity to light | 0 | 1 | 2 | 3 | 4 | 5 | 6 |
| Irritability | 0 | 1 | 2 | 3 | 4 | 5 | 6 |
| Sadness | 0 | 1 | 2 | 3 | 4 | 5 | 6 |
| Nervous/Anxious | 0 | 1 | 2 | 3 | 4 | 5 | 6 |
| Feeling more emotional | 0 | 1 | 2 | 3 | 4 | 5 | 6 |
| Numbness or tingling | 0 | 1 | 2 | 3 | 4 | 5 | 6 |
| Feeling slowed down | 0 | 1 | 2 | 3 | 4 | 5 | 6 |
| Feeling like "in a fog" | 0 | 1 | 2 | 3 | 4 | 5 | 6 |
| Difficulty concentrating | 0 | 1 | 2 | 3 | 4 | 5 | 6 |
| Difficulty remembering | 0 | 1 | 2 | 3 | 4 | 5 | 6 |
| Visual problems | 0 | 1 | 2 | 3 | 4 | 5 | 6 |
| Other | 0 | 1 | 2 | 3 | 4 | 5 | 6 |
| Total | | | | | | | |

## BALANCE ERROR SCORING SYSTEM (BESS)

### Balance Examination

This balance testing is based on a modified version of the Balance Error Scoring System (BESS). A stopwatch or watch with a second hand is required for this testing.

### Balance testing

*"I am now going to test your balance. Please take your shoes off, roll up your pant legs above ankle (if applicable), and remove any ankle taping (if applicable). This test will consist of three twenty second tests with different stances."*

(a) Double leg stance:

*"The first stance is standing with your feet together with your hands on your hips and with your eyes closed. You should try to maintain stability in that position for 20 seconds. I will be counting the number of times you move out of this position. I will start timing when you are set and have closed your eyes."*

(b) Single leg stance:

*"If you were to kick a ball, which foot would you use?* [This will be the dominant foot] *Now stand on your non-dominant foot. The dominant leg should be held in approximately 30 degrees of hip flexion and 45 degrees of knee flexion. Again, you should try to maintain stability for 20 seconds with your hands on your hips*

and your eyes closed. I will be counting the number of times you move out of this position. If you stumble out of this position, open your eyes and return to the start position and continue balancing. I will start timing when you are set and have closed your eyes."

(c) Tandem stance:

" Now stand heel-to-toe with your non-dominant foot in back. Your weight should be evenly distributed across both feet. Again, you should try to maintain stability for 20 seconds with your hands on your hips and your eyes closed. I will be counting the number of times you move out of this position. If you stumble out of this position, open your eyes and return to the start position and continued balancing. I will start timing when you are set and have closed your eyes."

**Balance testing-types of errors**
1. Hands lifted off iliac crest
2. Opening eyes
3. Step, stumble, or fall
4. Moving hip into > 30 degrees abduction
5. Lifting forefoot or heel
6. Remaining out of test position > 5 sec

Each of the 20-second trials is scored by counting the errors, or deviations from the proper stance, accumulated by the athlete. The examiner will begin counting errors only after the individual has assumed the proper start position. **The modified BESS is calculated by adding one error point for each error during the three 20-second tests. The maximum total number of errors for any single condition is 10**. If an athlete commits multiple errors simultaneously, only one error is recorded but the athlete should quickly return to the testing position, and counting should resume once subject is set. Subjects that are unable to maintain the testing procedure for a minimum of **five seconds** at the start are assigned the highest possible score, ten, for that testing condition.

Which foot was tested:    Left    Right
(i.e. which is the **non-dominant** foot)

**Condition    Total errors**

| | |
|---|---|
| Double Leg Stance (feet together) | of 10 |
| Single Leg Stance (non-dominant foot) | of 10 |
| Tandem Stance (non-dominant foot at back) | of 10 |

**Balance examination score** (30 **minus** total errors)    of 30

*Modified version of original assessment of postural stability (Guskiewicz, 2003), used with permission

# Resources

Centers for Disease Control and Prevention
http://www.cdc.gov/concussion/index.html

http://www.cdc.gov/concussion/pdf/TBI_returning_to_
school-a.pdf

Communique-NASP
http://www.nasponline.org/publications/cq/39/8/sport-
related-concussions.aspx

ESPN Video- *Life Changed by Concussion*
http://espn.go.com/video/clip?id=7525526&category
id=5595394

Nationwide Children's Hospital- *An Educator's Guide to Concussions in the Classroom*
http://www.nationwidechildrens.org/concussions-in-the-
classroom

REAP: A Sports Concussion Care Guide
http://www.sportsconcussions.org/REAP.html

REAP: Concussion Management Guidelines
http://www.rockymountainhospitalforchildren.
com/sports-medicine/concussion-management/reap-
guidelines.htm

SportsConcussions.org
http://www.sportsconcussions.org/ibaseline/

Sports Legacy Institute: Solving the Concussion Crisis
http://sportslegacy.org/

Upstate University Hospital- *Concussion in the Classroom*
http://www.upstate.edu/pmr/healthcare/programs/
concussion/classroom.php

Books

Cantu, R. & Hyman, M. (2012) Concussions and Our Kids: America's Leading Expert on How to Protect Young Athletes and Keep Sports Safe. Houghton, Mifflin, Harcourt.

Carroll, L. & Rosner, D. (2012). The concussion crisis: Anatomy of a silent epidemic. New York, NY: Simon & Schuster.